CANCER TREATMENT AND RESEARCH IN HUMANISTIC PERSPECTIVE

Steven C. Gross, Ph.D., is Professor of Psychology at Loretto Heights College, Denver, Colorado, where he has recently helped develop a college major in the field of Health and Wellness. As a Counseling Psychologist, he also works with the Department of Counseling Services at Loretto Heights College. In addition, Dr. Gross is the Medical Psychology Consultant to the Educational Institute of America and the New Family-Life Clinic. In the past, he has been an owner, Health Care Administrator, and Head of the Department of Social Services for a 250-resident medical rehabilitation center serving many cancer patients. Dr. Gross' current clinical interests in behavioral medicine are focussed on chronic pain, cancer rehabilitation, and infertility.

Solomon Garb, M.D., was a noted oncologist, pharmacologist, and cancer researcher. For ten years, he served as Scientific Director and President of the Medical Staff at the AMC Cancer Research Center and Hospital, Denver, Colorado. Dr. Garb was also Professor of Medicine at Colorado University Health Sciences Center, and Affiliate Professor of Clinical Pharmacology at Colorado State University, Fort Collins, Colorado. As a nationally recognized cancer research advocate, he often appeared as an expert witness before the United States Congress. He authored numerous books and articles on cancer and was Founder and Co-chairman of the Citizen's Committee for the Conquest of Cancer. Dr. Garb passed away of cancer while working on this volume.

CANCER TREATMENT AND RESEARCH IN HUMANISTIC PERSPECTIVE

Steven C. Gross, Ph.D.
Solomon Garb, M.D.

Editors

Foreword by R. Lee Clark, M.D.

Springer Publishing Company
New York

Copyright © 1985 by Springer Publishing Company, Inc.

Springer Publishing Company, Inc.
200 Park Avenue South
New York, New York 10003

85 86 87 88 89 / 10 9 8 7 6 5 4 3 2 1

Library of Congress Cataloging in Publication Data

Main entry under title:
Cancer treatment and research in humanistic perspective.
  Includes bibliographies and index.
    1. Cancer—Treatment. 2. Medicine—Philosophy. 3. Humanistic ethics. I. Gross, Steven C. II. Garb, Solomon. [DNLM: 1. Humanism. 2. Neoplasms—therapy. 3. Research. QZ 266 C2194]
RC270.8.C383   1985   616.99'4   84-20205
ISBN 0-8261-4760-7

Printed in the United States of America

This volume is dedicated to Solomon Garb, M.D.

Just as torches . . . grow pale and lose their brightness in the sun,
so intelligence, even genius, and beauty likewise, are eclipsed
and thrown into the shade by goodness of the heart.
[Schopenhauer]

We also remember the lives of Max Kivel and Nurit Kolodni,
individuals whose humanism far transcended their cancers.

The mind-body problem will never be solved by ignoring the troublesome factors, either those of spirit or of matter . . . . Traditional materialism and classical spiritualism both involve neglect of a vast wealth of human experience, including common sense and refined scientific knowledge. We cannot choose between materialism and spiritualism. We must have both.
[C. J. Herrick]

It is not the business of science to inherit the earth, but to inherit the moral imagination; because without that man and beliefs and science will perish together.
[Jacob Bronowski]

Freedom is what you do with what has been done to you.
[Jean Paul Sartre]

Contents

In Memoriam

Cancer research and treatment programs lost a good friend and one of their greatest allies with the passing of Dr. Solomon Garb. I always considered my relationship with Dr. Garb, which began in 1974 when I assumed the position of Director of the Division of Cancer Treatment of the National Cancer Institute, as very special. He was an activist. He felt very strongly about the need for a cancer program with balanced components of greater support for basic research and greater emphasis on the application of the results of basic research. He also realized instinctively that spanning both requirements is scientifically and politically sensitive. Accordingly, he kept his relationship to the leadership of the National Cancer Institute at a distance. He often told me that he was identified with some positions that were considered unpopular and therefore he preferred not to force them on me or the Institute by fostering the appearance of too close a relationship. He was a wise man and, despite this distancing, I felt close to him.

Dr. Garb was by training a pharmacologist and had good insights into cancer drug development. He was often the bearer of good scientific advice. On occasion we adopted suggestions made directly by him regarding the management of the drug development program. He received little credit for these ideas—again, by his own choice.

In reviewing his letters to the directors of the National Cancer Institute, correspondence that spanned the tenure of several before me, it became obvious that my own experience was not unique. He revealed himself to be a man of great breadth and a fine ability to reflect on events and ideas and to arrive at insights that added a new dimension to our understanding. There also are many instances of his coming to the defense of the cancer program, wading into the fray to ensure that his viewpoint was heard. The most notable instance of this was his recent defense of the philosophy of all-out treatment of cancer.

   As Co-chairperson of the Citizens' Committee for the Conquest of Cancer, he will be remembered for his tireless effort on behalf of cancer research and improving care for cancer patients.

                                        Vincent T. DeVita, Jr., M.D.
                                        Director
                                        National Cancer Institute

Foreword

In approximately 300 B.C., the Hippocratic school in Alexandria introduced a novel idea that changed the course of medical investigation and was responsible for eventual advancement of the knowledge of human anatomy, physiology, and diseases. This novel idea was based on the conviction that disease is a natural phenomenon, the causes of which lie within the human being or the immediate surroundings rather than with the gods or supernatural forces. It naturally followed that the human being was the "laboratory" and was to be studied, alive and dead, as the source of information regarding both normal and abnormal physical conditions.

Even with all of the advancement in the broad and specialized fields of medicine, there remains a sense of trepidation with the concept of "experimentation on human beings." All agree that the path to knowledge eventually leads to and through the human body; however, the degree of invasion and manipulation is under continuous scrutiny, challenge, and reevaluation, primarily because of a sometimes realistic distrust of both human nature and the drive of scientific fervor and ambition. The extreme proof of the validity of this distrust came with the knowledge of the atrocious, authorized experimentation perpetrated by Nazi physicians and scientists on captive human beings. The basic differences, of course, between this type of "experimentation" and legitimate experimentation are the essentials of (1) intent to help the patient who is voluntarily participating in the clinical trials and, if results are as positive as anticipated, to help countless other human beings also, and (2) in the case of healthy volunteers, intent to do no harm to them in exchange for their participation.

Few challenge the importance of eventual human experimentation after all that can be learned from other forms of life has been harvested and shared. Yet, are there unique situations in which so-called short-cuts can be justified? The essential ingredient in human experimentation must be compassion, but, as is true of any other human emotion, compassion is subject to interpretation.

As an example, we can examine the conflicting definitions of compassionate protection in the field of oncology. Without direct medical intervention, most patients with cancer (even "innocuous" skin cancer) will die, because our therapies are not sufficiently effective to control or eliminate widely spread metastases. Two of the three major therapeutic modalities—radiotherapy and chemotherapy— can be carcinogenic, toxic to normal cells, and life-threatening themselves. Nevertheless, oncologists hear hundreds of urgent pleas each day to "try anything that might work," that might extend life long enough for a possible future therapy with a more curative effect to be developed.

Oncologists, with their specialized training, wish to exercise their judgment to help these desperate people and wish for a sufficient degree of independence to try potentially useful new therapies. In the past, interpretation of compassionate protection has been different for oncologists than for federal employees of the U.S. Food and Drug Administration, whose responsibility it is to prohibit the use or marketing of any substance with potential harm to citizens, well or ill. Therein lies the quandary—tumoricidal drugs are harmful as well as helpful, so how can we protect as well as help patients with cancer? Both sides, the regulators and the physicians, want the same end result—healthy citizens. Their means of achieving the common goal sometimes have led to conflict. Except for the dying individual who wants to live, the controversy, which in reality is a series of checks and balances, is healthy and necessary to some degree. Generally, the best treatment is that given by a physician knowledgeable in the research horizons yet to be attained in the related field of medicine.

How do human beings find and accept norms except through knowledge of what the unacceptable extremes are? Quite naturally, imagination and previous experience can lead us close to norms without our actually having to become involved in the extremes. The danger in any human experimentation is that, although the initiating view is clear (benefit to humankind), the intellectual pursuit of the solution to the problem can become paramount and the participating patients themselves may become, in the minds of the experimenters, objects, means to an end rather than the means and the end.

The concept of the comprehensive cancer center has been to bring under one roof all aspects necessary to attack and solve the myriad problems caused by the numerous diseases included in the category of cancer. This has been an excellent philosophy for hastening the day when most of the basic problems will be solved. Cancer therapy is better than it has ever been; cancer research is more sophisticated and is yielding relevant information at an increasingly rapid pace; and cancer education and training is creating a growing number of individuals skilled at detecting, diagnosing, treating, and following up on patients who have cancer. As we get ever nearer to solutions that will prevent many cancers and prevent metastases after cancer develops, we have a tendency to become impatient that progress is not faster still. Success, for the first time, is in sight. There is inclination to overlook the very ageless, basic needs of every human being for love, patience, compassion, and protection—the cushions against vulnerability and physical and emotional pain.

For the oncologist with his or her eye on the light at the end of the scientific tunnel, today may just be another time period to be impatiently endured. But for each cancer patient, today is very precious, because it is perhaps one of the very few remaining ones, or it may be the very last today the patient will ever have. Even if the patient lives many months or years, some of the activities carried out in an impersonal research hospital environment may leave permanent scars that will mar all of the patient's remaining tomorrows.

We, in our scientific ardor to solve problems, must guard diligently against inflicting the deep wounds of indifference, the "unkindest cut of all."*

R. Lee Clark, M.D.
President Emeritus and System Professor
  of Surgery and Oncology
Professor of Surgery and Oncology
The University of Texas System Cancer Center,
  M.D. Anderson Hospital and Tumor Institute
Houston, Texas

*Shakespeare, William: *Julius Caesar*, Act III, Scene 2. (Part of a line spoken by Mark Antony following Caesar's assassination, speaking of the "friendship" between Caesar and Brutus, quoting Caesar when he realized that his friend, Brutus, participated in the assassination and delivered the "unkindest cut of all.")

Introduction

Few individuals remain personally or professionally unaffected by cancer. Cancer occurs in one out of every four persons in the U.S., directly involving two out of every three families. Cancer, therefore, is most certainly a scientific and humanistic problem of global concern, and nearly every physician, nurse, and allied health professional eventually will deal with the many difficult issues relating to cancer and its victims.

Our modern technological sciences and our advanced teaching centers provide wonderful and important information about the "structure," "function," and "treatment" of cancer, but they do little to prepare us to deal with the human issues that inevitably accompany the disease: "personal meanings," "quality of life," "ultimate purposes," and "consequences of decision."

Cancer literature traditionally has been divided into three artificially distinct and generally mutually exclusive content categories: (1) scientific research, (2) clinical treatment, and (3) humanistic, social, and moral issues. The present volume presents an overview of many of the common elements and interactions among these often polarized perspectives.

Because of the vastness of the topic, we have had to be selective; as a result, this volume is not a comprehensive textbook of cancer. Moreover, not all the opinions and values expressed by our contributing authors are shared by the editors. This book is designed to include highly respected authors whose personal value systems may lead them to differing conclusions. Perhaps the message in this diversity is simply that neither science nor moral philosophy nor human behavior can provide us with absolute certainties. Although disciplines and approaches vary, a humanistic concern and dedication to maintaining a high quality of life is shared by each contributor.

It is hoped that the topics discussed in this volume will lead to an expanded awareness of the effects of cancer on the patient and on the patient's family. The editors have sought to draw attention to "value," "responsibility," and "freedom" issues affecting cancer research and cancer treatment programs and to address the personal needs and struggles of the cancer professional and of those who wish to work with cancer patients in the future. The ultimate goal is to justify and clarify the need for a closer and co-equal relationship between humanism and science in cancer.

As a final note, we would like to thank Lea Gross and Richard Garb, whose help and support contributed greatly to the realization of this volume.

Steven Gross, Ph.D.
Solomon Garb, M.D.

Contributors

John W. Berg, M.D.
Department of Pathology and of Preventive Medicine and Biometrics, University of Colorado School of Medicine
Denver, Colorado

Thomas H. Budzynski, Ph.D.
Clinical Assistant Professor, University of Colorado Health Sciences Center; and Clinical Director, Biofeedback Institute of Denver
Denver, Colorado

Roger J. Bulger, M.D.
President, University of Texas Health Science Center, Houston, Texas
Formerly Executive Officer of the Institute of Medicine, National Academy of Sciences
Washington, D.C.

Barrie R. Cassileth, Ph.D.
Director, Division of Human Resources Research, University of Pennsylvania Cancer Center
Philadelphia, Pennsylvania

Benjamin L. Crue, Jr., M.D., F.A.C.S.
Director, New Hope Pain Center
Pasadena, California
Clinical Professor of Surgery (neurological), and Director, Section of Algology, Department of Neurosurgery, University of Southern California School of Medicine
Los Angeles, California

Yvonne Fotes
Mother of a terminally ill teenaged daughter
Rapid City, South Dakota

Hortencia M. Hornbeak, Ph.D.
International Cancer Research Data Bank Program, National Cancer Institute, National Institutes of Health
Bethesda, Maryland

Carl G. Kardinal, M.D.
Division of Hematology and Medical Oncology, Department of Internal Medicine, Ochsner Medical Institutions
New Orleans, Louisiana

Irwin H. Krakoff, M.D.
Director, Vermont Regional Cancer
Center; and Professor of Medicine
and Pharmacology, College of
Medicine, University of Vermont
Burlington, Vermont

Arthur S. Levine, M.D.
Special Assistant for Scientific Co-
ordination, Division of Cancer
Treatment, National Cancer Insti-
tute, National Institutes of Health
Bethesda, Maryland

Faye W. McNaull, B.S.N., M.P.H.
Assistant Professor, Duke Univer-
sity School of Nursing and the
Duke Comprehensive Cancer Cen-
ter
Durham, North Carolina

Daniel S. Martin, M.D.
Institute of Cancer Research, College of Physicians and Surgeons,
Columbia University, New York;
and Memorial Sloan Kettering Cancer Center
New York, New York
Chairman, Committee on Unorthodox Therapies, American Society
of Clinical Oncology

**Ronald W. Raven, O.B.E., T.D.,
M.D., F.R.C.S.**
Consulting Surgeon, Westminster
Hospital, and Consulting Surgeon,
Royal Marsden Hospital and Insti-
tute of Cancer Research
London, England
Chairman, Marie Curie Memorial
Foundation
Founder, The World Federation of
National Voluntary Cancer Care
Associations

Robert C. Sawyer, Ph.D.
Biochemistry, Catholic Medical Cen-
ter Cancer Research Laboratories
Woodhaven, New York

John H. Schneider, Ph.D.
Director, International Cancer Research Data Bank Program, National Cancer Institute, National Institutes of Health
Bethesda, Maryland

T. Flint Sparks, M.A.
Behavioral medicine consultant, and
psychotherapist in private practice
Denver, Colorado

James Stinnett, M.D.
Associate Professor of Psychiatry,
University of Pennsylvania School
of Medicine; and Director, Psychia-
tric Consultation Liaison Services,
Hospital of the University of Penn-
sylvania
Philadelphia, Pennsylvania

Robert L. Stolfi, Ph.D.
Department of Surgery (research),
Catholic Medical Center of Brook-
lyn and Queens
Woodhaven, New York

Bruce N. Strnad, Ph.D.
Director, Counseling Services, Co-
lumbia College
Columbia, Missouri

Dianne E. Tingley, Ph.D.
Deputy Director, International Can-
cer Research Data Bank Program,
National Institutes of Health
Bethesda, Maryland

Harold Y. Vanderpool, Ph.D.
Professor of the History of Medicine, The Institute for Medical Humanities, University of Texas Medical Branch
Galveston, Texas

J. W. Yarbro, M.D., Ph.D.
Professor of Medicine, University of Missouri-Columbia
Columbia, Missouri
Formerly Director, The Cancer Center Program of the National Cancer Institute (1972-1975)

CANCER TREATMENT AND RESEARCH IN HUMANISTIC PERSPECTIVE

I
Cancer Research
and Humanism

1

Cancer Research and the Development of Cancer Centers

J.W. Yarbro

The National Cancer Act was signed into law in December of 1971, and for the next four years there was an annual increase (above inflation) in the budget of the National Cancer Institute. For the first three years of this expansion, this author was responsible for the direction of the Cancer Centers Program. During this time it was this author's privilege to view multidisciplinary cancer efforts from a national perspective, and midway through the first decade this author's reflections on the impact of cancer centers on the academic community were published (Yarbro & Newell, 1976). Over 10 years have passed since the passage of the act; it seems appropriate to reflect, once again, on the complex relationships between cancer centers and academia. This author's viewpoint, of course, comes from years of involvement in the field of cancer, but it is impossible to isolate cancer from the larger political question of the evolution of the biomedical sciences. Let us go back, therefore, and pick up four historical threads, beginning respectively in 1896, 1910, 1938, and 1965.

The year 1896 was significant in cancer research for several events that shaped (some would say warped) scientific attitudes about cancer. It was in this year that research led to the establishment of a biological concept of cancer treatment, a concept that was in error but set the pattern for cancer treatment research for almost a century. Five uncontrolled clinical trials serve to illustrate how we were led astray.

In 1896, Beatson reported the efficacy of oophorectomy in "inoperable cases of carcinoma of the mamma" (Beatson, 1896). Because this work preceded the Bayliss-Starling concept of hormones, the isolation of estrogen from the ovary, and the Nobel Prize discovery by Huggins in 1940 of the efficacy of orchiectomy in prostate cancer, Beatson's observations of the *systemic* treatment of cancer were ignored for half a century. Yet this was the first demonstration of effective systemic treatment of cancer.

In 1896 Dr. W. B. Coley was at the midpoint of his five-year study of 140 cancer patients treated with Coley's Toxin, a bacterial product used for immunotherapy (Coley, 1893, 1898). Although his work was later to be branded quackery and outlawed by the medical profession, it was clearly the precursor of the recent immunotherapeutic trials with BCG and *C. parvum*. Unlike Beatson's work, Coley's was not ignored, but its lack of efficacy caused it to be discredited.

Also in 1896, Sir William Osler was preparing the third edition of his famous text on medicine. In discussing his experience with cancer treatment, he noted only one chemical, arsenic, that was useful in the systemic management of advanced cancer. It was not until the end of World War II that another toxic agent, nitrogen mustard, was used in the treatment of systemic cancer, although hydroxyurea, a currently accepted chemotherapeutic agent, had been discovered in 1869 (Dresler & Stein, 1869) and its pharmacologic effects shown in 1928 (see Kennedy & Yarbro, 1966). But arsenic was a weak anticancer agent and did not launch a massive search for other drugs, as did the work on nitrogen mustard.

Thus, at the turn of the century the systemic treatment of cancer did not show promise and it did not form a part of our conceptual framework of cancer management. But this significant decade of the 1890s, which saw the failure of systemic therapy, gave birth to a concept of cancer therapy that has dominated the field to the present day.

Beatson reported his success with oophorectomy at the midpoint of a decade of research by William S. Halsted at Johns Hopkins. It was Halsted who firmly established the concept of the sequential spread of cancer from local to regional to systemic. This was the conceptual framework that provided the rationale for the radical mastectomy and other "classic" cancer surgery techniques. Fisher and Gebhardt (1978) observed that this set the stage for an era of surgery which must be viewed as incredible in terms of both its longevity and its freedom from criticism. Halsted (1891, 1898) evaluated both conventional and super-radical operations to achieve regional control. We know today that his concept of metastasis was in error and that systemic spread of cancer cannot be controlled by regional therapy; but, at the time and for almost a century, this became the dominant theme of cancer treatment. It is only recently that controlled trials have demonstrated that simple excision of a breast cancer is as effective as radical surgery.

As the new year of 1896 was about to begin, the world read of the most dramatic discovery of all, and one that set the final thread into the tapestry dominating our concept of cancer treatment. On December 28, 1895, Röntgen reported his discovery of "eine neue Art von Strahlen"—a new kind of ray, later called the x-ray (Röntgen, 1895). Within three years, apparent cure of skin cancer was reported (see Kaplan, 1979). Subsequently, radiation therapy became a standard modality for the regional treatment of cancer.

As we entered the twentieth century, therefore, medical science had developed a concept of cancer (regional cancer precedes systemic spread) and two therapeutic modalities for the treatment of regional cancer (radical surgery and radiotherapy). All that remained (it seemed) was to integrate these tools properly to achieve a cure. But all too often in science we may become the prisoners of our preconceptions. In no field is this more true than in cancer (Kardinal & Yarbro, 1979). If the concept is wrong, the direction of research will be wrong. Not until the present decade have we been fully aware of how wrong our concepts were. The subtle point we missed was this: Surgery and radiation can indeed cure local cancer, but, as research in breast cancer has demonstrated, dissemination of cancer regionally and systemically are simultaneous, not sequential, events. Thus, a focus of attention on regional control diverted us from what we now perceive as the central issue: systemic treatment of micrometastases.

As the Halsted concept of cancer proceeded on a collision course with history, an event transpired that provided the cement to set in concrete the conceptual errors of the gay nineties. Our second thread began in the year 1910, when a schoolmaster from Louisville, Kentucky, presented a report that revolutionized medical education (and, more important, academic structure). Abraham Flexner's report served as the rationale for the reorganization of American medical schools along university (and, more important, departmental) lines. It converted medical schools from trade schools into academic institutions. It provided the academic environment for scholarship. It laid the groundwork for the transfer of the medical Mecca from Europe to America. And, unfortunately, it established a system of medical education so resistant to change, that errors of concept and curriculum remained in place long after common sense dictated otherwise.

Our new, "regional" concept of cancer, then barely a decade old, was set like a stone into this newly solidifying slab of concrete. Department structure became the cornerstone of medical education, creating both benefits and handicaps. The most critical, for this discussion, was that departments were assigned what amounted to jurisdiction over groups of patients. This had the effect of rendering clinical research unimodal: Surgeons tried to develop better operations, internists better drugs, and radiologists better machines, but each group worked largely with the patients assigned to its jurisdiction.

The third year of significance was 1938, when the National Cancer Institute (NCI) was created as the first of our present National Institutes of Health (NIH). From the beginning the NCI pioneered new ideas, including a massive peer-reviewed support for medical research that extended far beyond cancer to change the entire course of twentieth-century biomedical science (and provide a major component of the support for Flexner's departments which grew in strength with each dollar). Later, the NCI was the first institute to develop programs in large cancer research centers, massive controlled clinical-trials programs, and disease control programs. Federal funding converted medical schools to institutions in which research was commonplace and cancer research benefited along with all the rest. But as the NIH gradually emerged, a glaring conflict became apparent: The institutes did not follow the Flexnerian departments, but were based instead upon disease problems. Thus, Congress appropriated money to fight heart disease, cancer, and stroke, but these funds had to be divided among investigators structured along the Flexnerian lines of Medicine, Surgery, and Radiology.

Starting in 1938, then, the Flexnerian structure was placed in a strained configuration: The investigators were organized in accordance with the *tools* they used (drug, scalpel, x-ray), whereas the funds were allocated to solve *problems* that might require multiple tools.

The year 1965 was critical to this sequence of events. It was in this year that Medicare and other health legislation virtually eliminated the charity patient on which many medical school hospitals depended. Patient fees suddenly became a dominant factor in medical school budgets. From that time on, the medical school began to compete actively with its own graduates for the patients (and dollars) upon which both teacher and former student depended for their livelihoods. Within medical schools, furthermore, there was competition between departments for the patients each needed to survive. It was in the financial interest of each department to guard jealously those patients assigned to it by tradition.

By the time of the passage of the National Cancer Act the medical school structure had hardened into Flexnerian tradition: Research dollars reached an investigator through the department, patient fees reached the investigator through the department, and patients were assigned upon hospital admission to departments that everyone agreed had proper jurisdiction over their care and their access to new treatment modalities. Our "regional" theory of cancer, the Halsted concept, had become in due course an integral part of the system.

The attempt so far has been to describe the academic soil, or structure, admittedly from the bias of a cancer scientist. Let us turn now to a consideration of the seed, the cancer investigator with an idea. Investigators whose primary focus is cancer are by their very nature multidisciplinary in orientation because cancer is a multidisciplinary problem. (Discipline is used here in the Flexnerian sense, that is, based on the tools that are used rather than on the common body of biological knowledge needed to solve a problem.) Thus, the cancer scientists in Flexnerian academe must channel their natural instincts; they must say, "What question can we ask with the tools we are allowed?" rather than, "What tools do we need to answer the question that confronts us?"

The academic institution does not provide fertile soil for the seed of multidisciplinary inquiry. This is probably the reason why so many cancer centers developed as institutes outside of the academic structure.

In Europe, free-standing institutes have long been the rule rather than the exception, but our adaptation of Flexner's concepts (with all the obvious benefits) imposed a handicap on free-standing institutes. Such institutes simply were not in the "first class" academic tradition. The statistics on success are indisputable. The vast majority of cancer centers created outside of universities have failed. The cancer scientist is presented with a paradox: The academic climate, while hostile to centers, is essential for their ultimate success.

Perhaps it would be useful to select a noncancer biological problem to illustrate this paradox. Consider the interfaces between pediatrics, obstetrics, gynecology, and surgery. Set on our course by our belief in the dominant role of anatomy as a Flexnerian basic science, we continue to train young people in obstetrics and gynecology long after advances in knowledge make it far more rational to teach gynecology as a subspecialty of surgery and to train full-fledged obstetricians well versed in neonatology. Pediatrics has identified a body of knowledge, neonatology, that has far more in common with obstetrics than with the other aspects of pediatrics. Today there are centers where individuals experienced with high-risk pregnancies and complicated newborn management provide excellent care to mother and child and conduct research as a team. But, reflect for a moment on the tortuous training programs that must be followed by such investigators before they obtain the single body of knowledge required to become functional researchers. In biology we have learned that ontogeny recapitulates phylogeny, mandated by biological law; but, it is hardly mandatory that our training programs and our scientific organizational structure similarly reflect their tortuous historical origins.

What is suggested in this chapter is simply this: We in academe have not properly provided for the convergence of multiple established disciplines for the study of a single biological problem; we have failed to provide a functional academic structure for individuals who use the same body of knowledge on the same biological problem when that effort requires multiple tools. We pay a high price for this administrative gap. We do not, to use a phrase from military strategy, concentrate our forces. This fragmentation has led to less-than-optimal research design and poor coordination of patient care in our academic medical centers. This is as true for cancer as it is for other merging disciplines. Its origins can be traced directly to the Flexnerian concept of the discipline as a *tool.*

Surgery provides an example of ontogeny recapitulating phylogeny. The surgical specialties were defined at a time when anatomy dominated physiology, biochemistry, pharmacology, and the biology of disease. Once defined, these specialties have defied change. Radiology provides another example. The long and often bitter struggle to liberate therapeutic radiology from its phylogenic ancestor, diagnostic radiology, illustrates the cost of such change. Medical oncology, similarly, was initially "assigned" to hematology because several early conquests of systemic cancer occurred in patients "assigned" to hematological jurisdiction.

Indeed, most of the academic disputes in regard to cancer are jurisdictional disputes, a phenomenon academicians find amusing when labor unions are involved but see as deadly serious within medical schools. The very fact that most of the academic cancer controversy was jurisdictional should have provided a clue that our problem was organizational. That it did not illustrates the awesome power of tradition and vested interest in academe, in the very homeland of those who take pride in their ability to think new thoughts.

Halsted's theory was wrong, but so were many other theories whose challenge and change formed the steps to higher knowledge. The fatal mistake was setting Halsted's theory into an administrative and jurisdictional structure that permitted it to be challenged only by a better idea using the same tools. As subsequent research has shown, the challenge to Halsted required the use of a different tool.

Nor can Flexner be blamed. His concept of biomedical science within the university environment provided the key to the greatest flourishing of biomedical knowledge that the world has ever seen when coupled to the peer-reviewed federal grant support concept that began with the establishment of the NCI. Rather, it was the manner in which we in academe applied Flexner's principles to make departments the components of a completed structure rather than the foundations for the growth of new knowledge. We made departments into fiefdoms that resisted change. Consider the following memorandum, written to his dean by a professor charged with recruiting a center director for a major university:

> I do not think my recruiting efforts can be fruitful if every time I bring someone, the Chairmen mount the ramparts of their fiefdoms to repel the invader. [See Yarbro & Newell, 1976]

It was into this rigidly structured and change-resistant milieu, then, that the National Cancer Act thrust the concept of a multidisciplinary cancer center. The result should have been no surprise. There were really three major elements in the act: increased support for basic cancer research, multidisciplinary cancer research centers, and cancer control (or outreach from university to community for transmission of new knowledge). I have commented on the third aspect elsewhere (Yarbro, submitted for publication).

The first element was readily—indeed, eagerly—integrated into the university structure because the system was able to handle traditional grants. Such grants fit in reasonably well with established departmental autonomy; therefore, the act markedly increased the quantity and quality of basic research in cancer.

The second element, cancer centers, was not received so readily; in fact, centers were opposed from the beginning. As the guidelines for the cancer center program were being written, there was a clear vision of the kinds of programs that were intended to be supported. At the outset it was recognized that, if cancer centers were to have long-term viability and productivity, they would have to be developed in universities and become an integral part of the academic system. Several additional assumptions were inherent in these guidelines:

1. The state of the art in 1972 provided the capability for major progress in cancer research.
2. Some of that progress could be made by unidisciplinary research under support by traditional research grants; however, other progress required multidisciplinary research, that is, research into multimodal and alternative therapies.
3. Multimodal and alternate-modal therapy research would require a mechanism to bridge the existing jurisdictional (i.e., modal or departmental) mechanism for assigning patient responsibilities, since those responsible for care also determine what research will be done.
4. The cancer center should offer the potential to serve as the administrative mechanism for lowering existing barriers to multimodal and alternate-modal research.

Given such assumptions, then, the guidelines emphasized the importance of center autonomy that was parallel to the departmental autonomy that had so rigidly structured medical schools along departmental lines. This approach flew directly in the face of existing financial/status incentives that were operating to preserve a departmental structure that was largely historical in origin. The appeal was intended to be directly to deans and vice-presidents, over the heads of department chairmen, who, unless they happened to be oncologists, quite naturally would be motivated to a preservation of the status quo. The strength of the vested interest in the status quo was not minimized; on the contrary, every effort was made to maximize the reward for changing the system through such incentives as funds for new building construction, annual support budgets of highly flexible funds allocated similarly to existing departmental budgets, federal recognition as a "national comprehensive cancer center," and exclusive access to grant and contract support. Indeed, the package was designed to offer a complete department (or department equivalent), including space, budget, and grant programs. It was hoped, perhaps in vain, that existing faculty, in effect, would switch allegiance to this new administrative entity with senior institutional leadership support and bring their patients and expertise into common effort.

Three problems were encountered quite early in this process. The first was a miscalculation of the strength of the vested interests in the status quo. Most medical schools were not run by strong deans; rather, department chairmen had long since learned the strength of unity. Indeed, the preservation of an administrative structure that was largely an anachronism should have provided a clue to this.

The second problem had to do with how much a given institution needed the new funds. Those institutions already strong in research could obtain generous increases in their resources from the increased funding available for unidisciplinary research under the Cancer Act. They were far less likely, therefore, to be influenced to make the painful administrative changes than those institutions with less research talent.

The third problem was related to the nature of the review process. Reviewers, by their very nature, looked first at the quality of the research program of a potential center under review, without regard to the commitment of the institution to change from unidisciplinary to multidisciplinary research. Institutions strong in research consistently received priority scores superior to those weak in research, independent of compliance to the mandate for multidisciplinary programs.

These three problems operated together to produce a dilemma for those interested in encouraging multidisciplinary research: Institutions clearly dedicated to preserving the status quo tended to rank highest on the approved and funded lists, while those dedicated to multidisciplinary research tended to rank lowest. Yet, funding the unidisciplinary institutions reduced the power of the NCI to enforce the multidisciplinary guidelines on those institutions where a commitment to a new approach might be realized.

Furthermore, few seriously believed that the NCI would continue to receive the generous increases in funds needed to maintain the program (in fact, allowing for inflation, these increases continued for only four years). Thus, the name of the game, for the university, was to maximize short-term receipts and minimize long-term commitments. From the cancer point of view, we had a brief "window" in time (about five years) to accomplish a major change in university attitudes.

One minor controversy that deserves documentation related to the conversion from large block grants—"umbrella grants," in the slang of the time—to a mixture of "core grants" plus program grants. Originally, an entire center was funded by a single grant under the control of the center director. Under the "core grant" concept, the director controlled the core grant but each investigator and each team of investigators received individual peer-reviewed grants. The "umbrella grant" promoted multidisciplinary research because the empire-building tendency of a strong center director coincided with the intent of the centers program. The mixture of grants, on the contrary, promoted fragmentation because grants were divided between established departments. The official justification for the change was that "umbrella grants" were difficult to review because they were so large. This was no small consideration, because the peer-review process is the keystone of the entire NH system; to abuse it would bring discredit upon the very program NIH was working so hard to make acceptable. But, there were two additional underlying reasons for the change. First, the National Cancer Act placed a $5-million annual limit on center grants (this was interpreted to mean each grant, not an institutional limit on all center grants). Many large centers could not exist with such a limit, and it seemed better to change the terminology rather than ask Congress to change the law. Second, if the change to multidisciplinary research actually took place and centers became a way of life, the only way to bring centers into the "academic family" of departments was to insist on proper peer review of their investigators. The flexibility built into the "umbrella grant" (to make it attractive and functional), however, defeated the peer-review mechanism because it allowed the shift of funds to an investigator whose traditional grant was disapproved.

Thus the shift to the "core grant" concept was a calculated gamble; at one and the same time it reduced the chance of success, while standardizing the funding mechanism to make it more acceptable to the opponents of centers. The net result, viewed in retrospect, was a hodge-podge: Some centers were funded with no real hope they would ever become multidisciplinary; others were funded with no real hope that quality research would ever develop; and in most there was the near certainty that when the funds ran out the center would evaporate.

Another factor influencing the success of the centers program deserves mention (Yarbro, 1982). It is unlikely that proper implementation of the Cancer Control Program from the outset would have changed the end result, but the separation of "control" from "centers" at the NCI administrative level and the calculated efforts by the leaders of the Cancer Control Program to bypass existing centers in their programatic efforts certainly compromised the ability of cancer centers to achieve their goals. Of course, Cancer Control was not alone; each division of the NCI wanted to develop (and to some extent control) its own "team" of investigators and therefore there was a tendency to work around university centers rather than through them. This naturally strengthened the hand of university faculty opposed to the development of centers.

The central theme of the NCI centers programs was to develop centers with sufficient autonomy to make multidisciplinary clinical research a reality. While agreeing that centers would facilitate interaction between "clinicians who have heretofore lived in splendid departmental isolation," strong department chairmen at the time nonetheless condemned the autonomy that centers were achieving (Petersdorf, 1974). Not only were new organizational patterns not desired, such changes were considered highly unlikely. In 1975, 115 medical school deans ranked the emergence of new organizational disciplines as forty-seventh in a list of 54 changes likely to occur in the next 10 years (Keyes, Wilson, & Becker, 1975).

At times, university opposition to centers was bitter; at other times, it was amusing. On one occasion this author was privy to an early draft of a document from a prominent eastern school describing the principles under which a cancer center was being established. The differences between a center and a department were listed in the introduction. High on the list it was noted that a center, unlike a department, should be phased out when it ceased to perform a useful academic function. Needless to say, the draft was changed, but this Freudian slip gives us insight into the academic thinking of the time.

It is this author's thesis that the reasons for opposition to centers can be understood only by understanding the historical evolution of the existing clinical departments and the once logical, now archaic, assignment of patients to departmental jurisdiction. Consider, for example, lymphoma, cancer of the ovary, and small-cell cancer of the lung: Their anatomical differences pale into insignificance in comparison to the common biological body of knowledge required to design a successful research strategy for each. Multidisciplinary centers focus on the commonalities of all cancers, whereas our academic institutions, structured by historical tradition, focus on jurisdictional differences between patients.

The pattern of success and failure of different kinds of center grants, in retrospect, now makes administrative sense. Few would dispute that the most successful of the center grants were those funding multidisciplinary laboratory research. This author does not accept the notion that this occurred because the state of the art was, somehow, more "ready" for research progress in the laboratory than in the clinic (or that bench researchers are somehow better than bedside researchers). Having personally done both and viewed both extensively from a national perspective, this author is convinced that the success of the multidisciplinary laboratory research centers was due, quite simply, to the interchangeability of laboratory investigators among basic science departments and the lack of jurisdictional disputes in the laboratory as contrasted with the clinic. In spite of Flexnerian tradition, there are few jurisdictional research disputes among basic science departments. So long as a half-dozen department members teach a rudimentary course for medical students, the bulk of the faculty slots in a department may be filled by funded investigators doing whatever they choose. In this sense, biochemists, pharmacologists, microbiologists, and so forth are interchangeable and, indeed, they often are interchanged. This is not the case in clinical departments.

The second most successful type of center grant was that in which the multiple disciplines involved only one clinical discipline but with several laboratory disciplines. Examples of such grants might be those involving radiotherapy plus various laboratory disciplines or hematology plus various laboratory disciplines. Here, in this author's judgment, the success resulted from the fact that the patients (the necessary requirement for clinical research) were already assigned by the existing system to the jurisdiction of the one and only clinical discipline in the center.

The least successful type of center grant was that in which several clinical disciplines were involved. The larger the number of clinical disciplines, the larger the problem. There are, of course, a number of examples in which two clinical disciplines worked well together, but in each case there seemed to be two strong pillars of excellence (conveniently, one in each discipline) that held the program together across continuing academic barriers. Thus, individual cooperation could work in spite of the system, but, often, when one individual moved to another institution the cooperation ceased; that is, the system had not changed.

The one type of center grant that can be rated nearly a complete failure was the centerpiece of the National Cancer Act: the comprehensive cancer center. More time and effort and money went into this concept than any other, yet this was the least successful. With the exception of the three centers that were essentially comprehensive prior to the act (and these had evolved with only a minimal classic academic relationship), we can point to only three or four centers that evolved within medical schools to a level comparable to that envisioned at the outset. The reasons for the failure of the rest, as has been pointed out, are inherent in jurisdictional disputes over patients. But, the successes are so few that it is difficult to derive any general formula for success. Each was associated with the exceptionally strong leadership qualities of the center director, but leaders of comparable ability failed in other institutions. It is important to remember that the comprehensive center concept was rejected by academia in the face of multiple potential rewards, including federal recognition of excellence, designation of eligibility for exclusive access to special grants and contracts, the opportunity for regional leadership through the cancer control program, and (at the time) the potential for special treatment by health systems agencies. In spite of such inducements, the established patterns of patient jurisdiction changed very little.

Can we identify those factors that have changed patient jurisdiction? Several examples of such change may be cited: small-cell lung cancer, diffuse histocytic lymphoma, germ cell tumors. In each case, however, most of these reassignments have taken place only after research in a few pioneering institutions had demonstrated the futility of one modality and the efficacy of another. What is in need of emphasis is that this research progress was made only by those institutions in which the jurisdictional barriers already had been bridged in the research process. The lesson of this is clear: Where a different mode of therapy is required for progress, progress can be made only if patient jurisdiction is determined by a mechanism other than mode of therapy.

We are thus presented with a vicious circle: By historical tradition, patient jurisdiction is based on discipline; discipline is defined by the *tool* of therapy, not an academic body of related biological knowledge; thus, our traditions impair progress based on alternate-modal or multimodal therapy.

At the time of this author's departure from the NCI in 1975, it already was apparent that the centers program had fallen far short of its goal of establishing 15 new comprehensive centers as permanent academic units capable of fostering multidisciplinary research. Including the three preexisting centers, there were less than a dozen institutions where success seemed possible. (It is important to note that "success" is used here in terms of centers, not quality research, which under the centers program was supported well and was highly productive.)

Today, 10 years after the act, there are only three or four university based centers that can be said to have attained the originally envisioned goals and a few more where the outcome is still in doubt. For the most part, these have either formal oncology departments or departments-in-fact (though not in name). There are, fortunately, many more schools in which two or even three clinical departments have begun to work together and the level of collaboration of basic science departments has been substantially raised.

Though short of our original expectations, these achievements can be considered a fair beginning. There are many more opportunities today for new investigators to address a biological problem directly, not merely search for a question they may ask with the tools they are allowed; however, much remains to be done.

Some year ago, when this author was debating this issue with a dean, he asked, "What will you do with all those supertrained cancer specialists when we finally conquer cancer?" The answer was that if we were lucky enough and smart enough to conquer cancer, surely we would be able to figure out what to do with all those extra specialists. The real fear was, and remains, that, if we "institutionalize" oncology without making our academic system more open to change, then this present generation of revolutionaries, in their turn, may stand as a bulwark against the next generation, whose ideas will be needed as much then as ours are now.

References

Beatson, G. T. On the treatment of inoperable cases of carcinoma of the mamma: Suggestions for a new method of treatment, with illustrative cases. *Lancet*, 1896, *2*, 104-107, 162-165.

Coley, W. B. A preliminary note on the treatment of inoperable sarcoma by the toxin products of erysipelas. *Post-Graduate Medical Journal*, 1893, *8*, 278-286.

Coley, W. B. The treatment of inoperable sarcoma with mixed toxins of erysipelas and Bacillus prodigiosus: Immediate and final results in 140 cases. *Journal of the American Medical Associations*, 1898, *31*, 389-395, 456-465.

Dresler, W. F. C., & Stein, R. Über den Hydroxylharnstaff. *Justis Liebig's Annals of Chemical Pharmacology*, 1869, *150*, 242-252.

Fisher, B., & Gebhardt, M. C. The evolution of breast cancer surgery: Past, present, and future. *Seminars in Oncology*, 1978, *5*, 385-394.

Halsted, W. S. The treatment of wounds with especial reference to the value of blood clot in the management of dead spaces. *Johns Hopkins Medical Journal*, 1891, *2*, 255-314.

Halsted, W. S. A clinical and histologic study of certain adenocarcinomata of the breast: And a brief consideration of the supraclavicular operation and of the results of operation for cancer of the breast from 1889 to 1898 at the Johns Hopkins Hospital. *Annals of Surgery*, 1898, *28*, 557-576.

Kaplan, H. S. Historic milestones in radiobiology and radiation therapy. *Seminars in Oncology*, 1979, *6*, 479-489.

Kardinal, C. G., & Yarbro, J. W. A conceptual history of cancer. *Seminars in Oncology*, 1979, *6*, 396-408.

Kennedy, B. J., & Yarbro, J. W. Metabolic and therapeutic effects of hydroxyurea in chronic myeloid leukemia. *Journal of the American Medical Association*, 1966, *195*, 1038-1043.

Keyes, J. A., Wilson, M. P., & Becker, J. The future of medical education: Forecast of the Council of Deans. *Journal of Medical Education*, 1975, *50*, 319-327.

Petersdorf, R. G. Departments of medicine—1973. *New England Journal of Medicine*, 1974, *291*, 440-446.

Röntgen, W. C. Über eine neue Art von Strahlen. Erste mitteilung. *Sitzgsber Physikal-med Gesellschaft* (Würzburg), Dec. 28, 1895, 132-141.

Yarbro, J. W. Back to square one. Submitted for publication.

Yarbro, J. W., & Newell, G. R. Cancer centers: Their relationship to the academic community. *Journal of Medical Education*, 1976, *51*, 487-495.

2

The Ethics of Clinical Experimentation with Anticancer Drugs

Harold Y. Vanderpool

The ethical dynamics of adult oncology generally and the ethics of clinical drug experimentation on cancer patients specifically have received very little attention. This is true even though highly charged public controversies have occurred over the conducting of anticancer drug experiments,[1-7] and even though the few authors who have focused either on the ethics of clinical chemotherapeutic research[8] or on the care of cancer patients[9] have pointed to important and serious ethical problems and dilemmas. This is not to say that clinical oncologists who are conducting research lack an awareness of the ethical dimensions of their work. They can, and sometimes do, speak at length about certain ethical issues. Occasionally and briefly, ethical issues also are discussed in articles within specialty journals which otherwise focus on technical and scientific analysis.[10-12] Sometimes these discussions are defensive,[13] and sometimes they focus more on problems created by "overzealous" ethicists and a bureaucratic stifling of research than on poignant and painful dilemmas faced by physicians, patients, and family members.[14] The important ethical issues within experimental oncology need to be identified, scrutinized, and discussed widely and publicly.

The purpose of this chapter is to examine the thought and actions of clinical oncologist–researchers in the light of the discipline of ethics. This chapter will characterize and discuss certain ethical dilemmas within experimental chemotherapeutic oncology with the hope that further interest and open exchange will occur. In order to accomplish this, we first shall seek empathetically to describe in some detail the values, thinking, and activities of oncologists who are conducting clinical experiments with chemotherapeutic drugs; second, to speak about ethics as a discipline of inquiry; and, third, to evaluate critically the world of oncological research in light of the discipline of ethics. Put simply, this chapter will look at experimental clinical oncology through the lens of ethics in order to discover how chemotherapeutic drug research might be conducted in conformity with ethical patterns of reasoning. We will focus on ethical issues involving competent adult patients and draw on the opinions, convictions, and judgments of a wide variety of persons.

The World of Chemotherapeutic Research

Given the variety of influential values that humans may have and the way those values are related to sensible patterns of thought and action, it is utterly necessary to understand the realities and value orientations of persons and institutions (including physician-researchers in cancer centers) in order to determine the role and status of moral values. Are ethical principles prioritized over other values? If not, what other values displace or compromise these ethical values, and why? How would an honoring of ethical values affect the behavior and value priorities of certain social groups—in this case, oncologists who are doing experimental research? These are fundamental questions that cannot be answered without an awareness of the "realities" and value priorities of the group under investigation.

Few physicians—and, behind them, all too few medical ethicists—have recognized the importance of identifying and displaying the value priorities of medicine. Those who have attempted to understand the value system of which they are a part have been able to highlight what actions and policy guidelines are necessary in order to give priority to ethical values and principles.[15] Without this awareness, medical and other professionals may be exceedingly well meaning and show little or no malice toward their patients, yet be so molded and influenced by the organizational realities and value dynamics of the institutions in which they work that they nonetheless act unethically.[16] These perspectives and possibilities inform this chapter's discussion.

The value system of clinical oncologist-researchers is composed of at least nine ingredients, all representing areas deserving far more detailed research and investigation. These ingredients are: (1) general rates and cures of cancer, (2) certain characteristics of chemotherapeutic research, (3) morbidity factors, (4) governmental and institutional efforts to effect cancer cures, (5) the roles and loyalties of oncologist-physician-researchers, (6) the roles of institutional review boards (IRBs), (7) the responses of patients, (8) the reactions of family members, and (9) the traditions of cancer cure. This chapter will note how these ingredients reflect certain fundamental values that represent an intact and sensible pattern of thought and action. The first six items will be discussed briefly in this section, and all nine will be addressed later within the context of ethics.

Rates and Cures of Malignant Neoplasms

Ever since the late 1930s, Americans have become increasingly aware of the degree to which malignant neoplasms have been a major cause of death. The latest statistical evidence indicates that deaths due to cancer are second only to those caused by various heart diseases. In 1978, approximately 400,000 Americans, or 20 percent of those who died, succumbed to cancer. This is compared to 730,000, or 37 percent, who died from heart diseases. At the present time, almost four times as many persons die of malignant neoplasms than from automobile, industrial, and other accidents. Death rates from cancer were more than 11 times greater than those from diabetes mellitus, and 18 times greater than those caused by acts of homicide.[17] These frightening mortality rates lie at the root of all efforts to overcome the ravages of malignant neoplasms.

Fortunately, due to the discovery of surgical, radiological, and chemotherapeutic procedures, cancer is not always lethal. Approximations of cure rates drawn from selected sources present these data in the following terms: Of an estimated one million Americans who presented with new cases of cancer in 1977, approximately one-third of these had malignancies on the skin or cervix that were curable; another 40 percent of the remaining 700,000 were treated successfully with some combination of surgery, radiation, and chemotherapy; of the remaining 42 percent (420,000), a first group of 250,000 persons had serious, inoperable neoplasms with distant metastases. It has been estimated that 11,000 of these were cured by chemotherapy alone and another 47,500 had their lives prolonged for at least a year.[18] A second group of 170,000 persons was likely to develop recurring tumors after surgery. Some 15,100 of these persons showed some response to chemotherapeutic drugs[18]; that is, their cancers shrank and/or their lives were prolonged.

The majority of the 11,000 persons who are cured every year by chemotherapy are cured of some 12 types of malignancies, including acute lymphocytic leukemia in children, Hodgkin's disease, and testicular carcinoma. The rates of life prolongation for the 47,500 patients with inoperable neoplasms also are cancer specific. For example, life can be prolonged for some 50 percent of those persons diagnosed with small-cell carcinoma of the lungs. The 15,100 of the approximately 170,000 patients or patient-subjects who are at high risk for a recurrence of cancer can or may respond to chemotherapeutic agents if these are administered at "optimal" dosages. Optimal dosages are defined by dose, dose schedule, and duration of treatments in order to maximize killing of cancer cells without permanently destroying normal ones.[19]

Again, these rates of benefit are cancer specific and, although experts disagree on the numbers affected, response rates are approximately as follows: from 20 percent to 40 percent of the 35,600 patients with breast carcinoma respond to optimal doses of chemotherapeutic agents. These response rates are less efficacious if optimal doses cannot be administered because patients are too weak or develop early toxic responses. Another 20 percent of the approximately 4,600 persons with rectal cancer will have their lives prolonged another 47 months if they receive two chemotherapeutic drugs and radiation after surgery,[18] and perhaps 5 percent to 10 percent of those with colon carcinoma or melanoma experience anticancer responses from chemotherapeutic drugs.[18]

Oncologist-researchers often rely on these rates to justify their procuring research funds and their great need to experiment on human subjects. For example, several authors have argued that the $500 million invested in chemotherapeutic research since 1955 has been well spent because it has led to the cure of some 11,000 persons per year (most of these young patients). These authors calculate that during their lives these 11,000 persons will pay $240 million in federal taxes and earn $1.6 billion in wages.[18] Furthermore, these same funds have made it possible to prolong the lives of another 47,500 patients on average for one year. This results in an extra 47,500 "person years of life annuality".[18] Experimental research is thus often justified because of its quantitative benefits as measured by dollars spent and returned and "person years" produced.

This quantitative justification of research is given further credence by comparing how much progress has been made over time. Compared with the fact that there were almost no usable anticancer drugs 30 years ago, chemotherapy has "added immensely to the success trends in cancer treatment."[19:618] Consider, for example, the dramatic changes in survival rates that have occurred for one specific malignancy. Whereas only 20 percent of those with testicular cancer could have their lives prolonged in 1960, and only half of these could expect to live disease-free lives, some 70 percent of those with testicular cancer now can expect to experience complete remissions, and the majority of these will remain disease free.[18]

Characteristics of Chemotherapeutic Research

Incremental progress against cancer through chemotherapy research has been made possible because various types of chemicals have been discovered that will destroy cancer cells faster and more effectively than they will destroy other cells and organs in the human body. In order to accomplish this "seek and destroy mission," these chemicals are necessarily strong and toxic. They produce pain and sickness and sometimes death. This gets to the essential problem of the subspecialty of oncology: Physicians and cancer patients have to decide when to seek cures and life prolongation in the face of sickness and the fact that cancer, for thousands of patients, is indeed "lethal if left untreated."[1]

Clinical experimentation on anticancer drugs is based on the hypothesis that better cure rates can be attained as new chemical agents are found and/or fresh combinations of new and already approved ("standard") drugs are discovered. Chemotherapeutic experimentation is being conducted for the purpose of discovering, and scientifically measuring, the effects of new drugs and fresh combinations of drugs in order to enhance cure rates while minimizing death, morbidity, and injury.

In order to accomplish these goals, chemotherapeutic research is staged according to three "phases," each of which raises special dilemmas. Phase I represents the first stage of research on humans after certain chemicals have been found to destroy cancers in animals, especially forms of leukemia in mice. This phase of research is set up so as to do the least amount of harm to humans, as these chemicals are first tested on animals before they are moved up to further phases of analysis and, hopefully, to curing. Up until 1977, some 500,000 chemicals of many varieties and from all over the world had been tested on leukemic mice for their anticancer effects.[20] Only about 50 of these chemicals were being moved toward human clinical trials in 1977, with 13 of this group designated as "best drugs" for possible testing in humans.[20] By 1981, approximately 40 drugs were judged to be "effective in treating cancer."[1]

After selected chemicals are identified as most effectively shrinking or destroying mouse tumors, they are tested in monkeys and dogs for their toxicity levels before they are tested on humans. They are tested primarily for their toxic effects on the blood and the gastrointestinal tract. Dogs have been found to be approximately 85 percent accurate as indicators for blood toxicity and 92 percent accurate for gastrointestinal complications.[20] Since experience has shown that chemotherapeutic agents are most effective when they are highly toxic, these agents must be carefully administered to humans in order to determine what levels, sequences, and durations of dosages humans can stand. These are called "optimal" dose levels, and, in order to discover what these are, oncologist–researchers must increase dosage levels gradually in phase I trials until some optimal level of toxicity and hoped-for benefit is achieved. There is much debate and disagreement over the degree to which these trials do or do not offer benefits to their human subjects.

The possible benefits and harms of newly discovered experimental drugs are difficult to assess because little is known about the metabolic and biochemical effects and activities of these agents.[20] In general these chemicals are discovered not by "the results of rationally based research synthesis programs," but as "the products of empirical screening" in mice, then dog, and then human systems.[20:613] This is why these chemical agents have to be tested in numerous combinations (sometimes discovered to be lethal), on numerous types of cancers, and even must be shown to be "successful" in four or five similar patient populations before their effects are understood more accurately.[20,18] This is also why some of the drugs are discovered to have devastating cardiovascular, renal, and other effects after they have been used for months and even years.[3,4,21,22]

Phase II trials involve administering these chemicals, according to the approximate dosage levels defined by Phase I studies, to groups of patients with similar types and severities of malignant neoplasms. Since it has been discovered that some chemicals affect certain types and stages of cancer far more than others, it is necessary to experiment with a single protocol on several populations of patients with various types of malignant neoplasms. This explains why the National Cancer Institute (NCI) approves of further tests for "best-rated" chemicals, even when these are found to be ineffective on some cancers and/or shown to be highly toxic for patients with these cancers.[3,4,18]

The chances for being harmed in Phase II are somewhat less than in Phase I, while the possibilities for benefit are somewhat greater. The chances for harm are lessened because Phase I tests have already determined maximally tolerable doses, and by using these dose schedules it is expected that these levels can be accepted by the human body. Nevertheless, possibilities for harm still exist and are common because the potent "optimal" levels, sequences, and numbers of doses are refined in Phase II trials as the drugs are administered to more patients and investigation on human pharmacology is undertaken. Newer, less-tried agents are especially risky and possibly toxic.[8] The possibilities for benefits also are greater in Phase II than Phase I because the populations of patients being tested are being studied expressly in order to see if the new drug will have an impact on their particular type and stage of neoplasm.

Although combined statistics are lacking, it appears that the possibilities for benefit are nevertheless "limited" in Phase II. They are limited because a given chemical (1) may not destroy or retard the growth of the specific cancer being studied, (2) may have little or no impact on advanced-stage cancers, and (3) may not improve the condition of a specific individual even though the chemical being investigated has been shown to have a "statistically significant" effect for the cancer that this individual has.

Phase III is less controversial with regard to possible harms and benefits. Having been screened for their toxicity and shown to be therapeutically effective on certain types of cancers, investigative chemicals are compared with standard therapies in Phase III. Nevertheless, harm–benefit ethical concerns still exist, depending upon the proven or suspected levels of effectiveness of new versus old chemotherapeutic agents.

There is yet another category, known as combination therapy. Much of the research now being done in all three of these research phases—particularly in Phase II and Phase III—involves administering newer, "best drugs," as well as standard agents, in different combinations and sequences. Combination therapy became popular after 1963, when it was discovered that survival rates for acute lymphocytic leukemia could be improved by varying the order and dose level of drugs that already were known to be useful as single agents in the control of leukemia. Between 1963 and 1975 this research on combination therapy increased the median survival of these patients from 24 to 46 months.[20] Similar changes were observed for survival in Hodgkin's disease and breast cancer, and these data have become the basis for a host of new experimental regimens.[20]

Several important features of cancer research are brought out by these observations. First, even as combination or multidrug therapies offer promises of benefit, so also do they give rise to a new set of possible harms, because, once these drugs are combined, they sometimes negate each other's effectiveness, sometimes create new toxicities, and sometimes enhance the toxicity of any other agent with which they are used. Numerous dangerous interactions have been identified and listed.[20] Multidrug regimens, therefore, must pass through all the phases of experimental trials before they can be proved to be either "safe" and/or effective.

Second, combination therapy greatly expands the number of trials that must be conducted in order to show which combinations are effective, which are ineffective, and which are lethal. If 20 promising drugs are investigated two at a time, 380 types of trials must be created for any single type of cancer. Twenty drugs used in combinations three at a time would give rise to 6,840 such trials.[20] With varying doses and schedules and different tumor types, the number of possible trials quickly becomes unmanageable.

Finally, reliance on combination therapy indicates that oncologists' hopes for achieving cure and life prolongation with these drugs are modest. Most oncologist-researchers do not expect to see great breakthroughs with existing drugs or the discovery of one or more miracle chemicals. The great majority of present experimental protocols involve hopes of improving incrementally the numerically modest statistics that have been outlined previously.[18] Nevertheless, chemotherapists are excited and enthusiastic when even incremental changes are discovered, for this represents both a personal and a group advance in the face of a long-standing war against cancer.

Morbidity Factors

We have noted how death or mortality rates often are used to justify the funding of all types of cancer research, as well as chemotherapeutic drug experimentation. In addition to mortality rates, oncological research also is predicated upon the desire to alleviate some of the sickness, pain, and suffering (morbidity) that accompany cancer. Descriptions of cancer over centuries of history graphically portray its morbid effects—the pitiful suffering of women with breast cancer; the racking pain, weakness, and bloody fluxes of men with prostate cancer; the inexorable, slow, wasted deaths of those who cannot digest food because of stomach neoplasms. Dying at home from cancer is often far from a peaceful, serene sharing of time and experience with families. Oncologists therefore feel that they are "benefiting" their patients with new drugs and drug combinations which may alleviate, for example, some of the pain and pressure of inoperable neoplasms that have aggressively invaded surrounding tissues and organs.

Yet, the chemotherapeutic drugs that are administered and/or experimented with also cause suffering and injury; and these morbidity effects must be considered in assessing the harms and benefits involved in home dying, palliative care, or becoming enrolled in experimental protocols. With respect to experimental drugs, the serious, sometimes life-threatening reactions of the human body to chemotherapeutic agents often are referred to as "side-effects."[1] It is more accurate, however, to view these effects as the "normal mechanisms of action" of these drugs.[20] Measurably and predictably, these chemicals have powerful effects on cancerous cells and organs of the human body, even though by definition and purpose they are targeted toward cancer cells.

What are some of the morbid effects of chemotherapeutic agents? Even though each drug creates its own series of reactions in the human body, nearly every major type of chemotherapeutic drug also produces nausea and vomiting, sometimes "violent and prolonged."[19,23] They also frequently produce painful ulcerations in the mouth and the gastrointestinal tract,[23-25] often cause alopecia or hair loss, especially on the scalp,[25,26] and cause patient-subjects to feel weak and exhausted.[19,25] Some of these chemicals also give rise to burning pain, especially in the hands and feet,[24] skin rashes and discolorations,[26] severe liver damage,[19] kidney damage,[21] irreversible heart damage,[22] lung damage,[27] mental abnormalities,[3,19] and even cancer itself, especially acute nonlymphocytic leukemia.[19]

When these problems become particularly severe, they are considered "dose-limiting." For example, the vomiting, ulcers, and appetite loss caused by methotrexate are so great that its dose level is limited even though organs of the body could endure higher dosages, and higher dosages might destroy more cancer cells.[19,28] Furthermore, the nausea and vomiting caused by many chemotherapeutic drugs are not affected greatly by standard antiemetic drugs— hence the interest by oncologists and the press concerning the use of marijuana for these symptoms.[19]

It must be emphasized that each chemical has to be looked at separately for its morbidity effects, especially its effects on internal organs. The various effects of some of the most important experimental agents have been charted.[19] Some chemicals like 5-Fluorouracil (5-FU) result in nausea (78-90%), vomiting (50-60%), ulcerations (63-70%), and diarrhea (34-85%) at therapeutic dose levels, yet seldom cause total hair loss.[19] Adriamycin causes hair loss in almost all patients (which will grow back in two to five months), ulcerations (70-100%), and has caused acute kidney failure and congestive heart failure.[19,21,22,26]

The deliberate, phase-controlled investigation of these drugs is designed to discover which side-effects will occur in order to choose dosage levels that control toxicity. Some oncologists have characterized these effects as "temporary, predictable, and manageable" if skilled experimenters carefully monitor patient-subjects.[18] Nevertheless, certain levels of morbidity, sometimes severe morbidity, are being sought[1]; and the "price required for success" is sometimes high, with the ultimate, nonfatal response being the development of a second malignancy.[19]

Governmental and Institutional Efforts

The first, full-scale "war on cancer" was declared in 1971, when President Richard Nixon signed legislation creating the National Cancer Program. Cancer research quickly developed some of the characteristics and dynamics of big business as the $190.4 million allotted in 1971 was increased to nearly $1 billion by 1980.[29] Forty-four percent of the amount spent in 1980 was used to sponsor the experimental work conducted by many investigators in major hospitals and health centers across America. Research grants have been assigned on a competitive basis by peer-review committees that fund the experimental research of the most promising and/or well-established investigators. Significant amounts of additional funding have been allotted for training programs and construction; and between 1971 and 1981 a number of major cancer centers were established in which various subspecialties within research and cancer treatment were consolidated.

Along with these developments, cooperative oncology groups have emerged that approve, oversee, and gather data on much of the chemotherapeutic research being conducted. The authority and actions of these groups deserve special scrutiny and raise issues that are beyond the scope of this chapter.

In addition to these notable nationwide developments, the mass media have sustained a climate of favorable opinion and excitement over the possibility of discovering new miracle drugs for cancer cures. In keeping with a long-standing American infatuation with science and technology, reporters for television, newspapers, and popular journals regularly tell how scientists have discovered how new chemicals can either cure tumors in mice or prove themselves effective on human cancers. The public discussion over the relatively nontoxic drug Interferon illustrates this excitement. Millions of dollars worth of Interferon have been purchased in the last several years by the American Cancer Society, from drug companies that invested heavily in its production.[30] In the summer of 1979 alone, the NCI announced that it would buy $9 million worth of Interferon for further investigation. Aware of these developments, *Time* magazine depicted a droplet of Interferon on its front cover, billing it as the big, exciting, possibly miraculous IF drug.[30] In spite of these expenditures and this media frenzy, Interferon now is assessed by some oncologist-researchers as "disappointing" with regard to its effectiveness as an anticancer drug.

The work of oncologist-investigators thus is supported by general notions of scientific and biomedical progress, by hopes for miracle cures, and by strong economic pressures and incentives. Chemotherapeutic experiments are part of a national campaign to help overcome the menace of cancer. This work generally is regarded as contributing to the common good, and, in order for it to continue, numerous clinical experiments must be conducted and thousands of research subjects must be enrolled.

Despite widespread hope and enthusiasm regarding chemotherapeutic experimentation, heated public criticisms and controversies have begun to emerge. In October 1981, for example, the *Washington Post* ran a series of articles by Ted Gup and Jonathan Neumann on the NCI's experimental drug program. Gup and Neumann alleged that these experiments are often painful, lethal, impersonal, and illegal and that cancer researchers sometimes treat research subjects like "guinea pigs."[3-6] Vincent DeVita, the director of NCI, responded with a critique and disclaimer to Gup and Neumann, charging that they had "a tragic lack of understanding of cancer treatments and the National Program, which is designed to discover more effective cures."[1] DeVita and other oncologists not only have sought to explain the purposes and defend the morality of these experiments,[1,7] but also have maintained that Gup and Neumann conducted their research insensitively and unethically.[7] These disputes dramatize the necessity of open and thorough scrutinization of the ethics of chemotherapeutic research.

Roles and Loyalties of Researchers

Oncologist–physician–researchers are highly skilled specialists who are called upon to perform several roles that presuppose diverse loyalties and values. Their active involvement with chemotherapeutic research on local, regional, national, and international levels presupposes commitments and loyalties to the national campaign against cancer, to the expansion of scientific knowledge regarding how cancers develop and affect humans, to academic peers who review and conduct clinical experimentation, and to personal career advancement and reputation. As participants and sometimes leaders in academic medicine, these specialists also are expected to value the fundamental goals of each medical center, namely, the general importance of research; of teaching and training medical students, residents, and fellows; and of providing effective patient care.

More than 50 years ago the well-known Boston physician, Richard Cabot, became convinced that dedicated physician-researchers could honor and harmonize their moral obligations.[31] However, some investigators are less than optimistic about the harmonizing of diverse value commitments. Sociologists have observed, for example, how these values often conflict because of the organizational demands and priorities of the research-oriented health science center. They have indicated how individual patients may be neglected, injured, and ethically wronged because they are given a low status in the actual value priorities of these institutions and sometimes are caught in the cross-fire of value conflicts between different groups of medical professionals.[16]

The pressures on and possibly conflicting values of oncologist-researchers cannot be minimized and discounted. Some cancer specialists have asserted publicly that these pressures and divided loyalties lead to a certain amount of coercion and exploitation of patients.[8] This problem sometimes occurs, for example, when chemotherapists in research-oriented medical centers exert pressures on residents, fellows, and peers to procure a high percentage of signups for IRB consent forms—with acceptance rates of 80 percent to 90 percent not uncommon. These medical care and researching teams also may discuss and propose specific methods for achieving high percentages of signups.

Finally, it must be remembered that physician–researchers are human, too; that is, they are involved personally and psychologically with the successes and failures of the treatments they offer. Although the psychological dynamics of this involvement have not been investigated, it seems possible that some oncologist-researchers rely on experimental research as a partial relief from the helplessness and the involved anguish they feel when their patients have to suffer and often die.[8] Many, understandably, are excited by the discovery of more effective cures,[7] and it is possible that this excitement partially compensates for the "loss" of many patients and serves as a factor in enrolling severely ill patients on research protocols.

Institutional Review Boards

Oncologist–investigators are required to work closely with IRBs, which perform several functions. These include assisting researchers in writing protocols, protecting human subjects from harm, influencing the development of institutional research policies, and serving as mediators among the patients, physician, and hospital when patients feel that they may have been harmed.[15] With respect to protecting patients, IRBs are commissioned to assess accurately the possible harms (risks) and benefits of each experimental project or protocol. The latest regulations for IRBs state that, when the risks involved are judged as more than minimal (defined as the types of risks persons take every day in their ordinary lives), IRBs are required to see that these risks are set forth clearly—along with possible benefits—on informed consent forms. These forms must be signed by patients before they can become the subjects of any phase of drug experimentation.[32,33]   These procedures are designed both to protect subjects from undue harm and to make sure that these subjects have the right to decide when they do or do not wish to participate in "at-risk" research.[32] Recent articles have emphasized that IRBs have been effective in controlling harmful and dangerous research.[32,33]

The purposes and contributions of IRBs have been developed over time by a number of regulative bodies and commissions. A processing of each research protocol through local IRBs may take considerable time and frequently raises disputes between researchers and those who are responsible for seeing that federal regulations are followed. Like physicians from other medical specialties, several oncologist-investigators have written that they are overburdened with the bureaucratic red tape spawned by "the current atmosphere of regulation," which they feel stifles innovative scientific progress.[14] These critics recognize that ethical screening is "desirable and necessary" in order to prevent abuses from occurring, but they resist bureaucratic probing by "Big Brother."[14] In the place of regulations, these critics of bureaucracy have called for general ethical guidelines and values that all conscientious investigators will abide by.[34] Certain utilitarian ethicists wholeheartedly agree with this minimal-rule, laissez-faire stance toward the conducting of human experimentation.[35] In short, while many oncologist–researchers have learned to live with IRBs, they are critical of excessive over regulation and probing, are trustful that most investigators will conduct their research in ethically conscientious ways, and genuinely believe that the ethical traditions of Western medicine should be known, appreciated, and reaffirmed.

Summary

This survey of the "real world" and values of clinical oncologist–researchers indicates that this is a tradition of thought and action with its own integrated pattern of values and practices. This tradition values its accomplishments as contributing to the great human war against cancer, helping to cure disease and prolonging human life in the face of great suffering and loss of life. It is a tradition of research that gradually has improved cure and life-prolongation rates by conducting numerous clinical experiments with the cooperation of thousands of research subjects. These research subjects are greatly appreciated and often admired and agonized over. As one oncologist-researcher recently remarked, they are appreciated for "contributing something very important to the future; they're being heroes." This is a tradition, finally, that seeks to balance care for patients and their families with teaching responsibilities, the expansion of medical knowledge, the building of cancer centers, competition for grants, and professional ambitions.

These values and convictions make sense psychologically, professionally, and morally to those who function within this value system. Indeed, there is a certain rugged and heroic character to this tradition of therapy and experimentation. It trains those within it to live every day with tough, painful, and complicated decisions; and it has managed to maintain a degree of optimism in the face of gradual successes that have required great amounts of work and the witnessing of the suffering and deaths of many cancer-ridden patients and have been accompanied by the demands of regulatory review organizations and by increasing degrees of public unrest.

Ethics As a Discipline

Ethics sometimes is equated falsely and uncritically with personalized concern, compassionate counseling, noble ideals, and even prudent, common-sensical action.[36] Although certain fundamental moral principles may be shown to include some of these concerns and ideals, the essential ingredients of human morality should be viewed as derived from a disciplined, rational investigation of principles that are coherent and defensible in the light of the character and dynamics of human existence. Individuals and groups can and do seek to justify the morality of their actions by a host of presumptions and arguments. Those who proceed from the discipline of ethics "tease out" all presumptions and arguments concerning human morality and critically scrutinize these for their logical coherence and validity. Out of this discipline certain general ethical principles have been discovered upon which reasonable persons can agree, principles that even strangers will want to follow because they seem reasonable and necessary.

Two modes of ethical reasoning that pervade discussions or research ethics are called, respectively, *prima facie* ethics and respect-for-person ethics. These two modes or models of ethical reasoning each are predicated upon an aspect of life and consciousness that enables humans to function and flourish as "persons," that is, as self-aware, reflective creatures who are responsive to others. Let us examine each of these in turn.

Prima Facie *Ethics*

This model of ethics assumes that our becoming and flourishing as human beings is dependent upon our having been incorporated into a human community that is able and willing to sustain and nurture us according to Van Melsen. Regardless of their particular beliefs and habits, communities that foster awareness, knowledge, and well-being adhere to certain basic moral prescriptions and prohibitions. These principles can be, and are, called the moral prerequisites of human communities, and they include acting benevolently (beneficence); refraining from stealing, killing, and other acts of maleficence; telling the truth (veracity); maintaining certain levels of justice; and expressing gratitude. These moral norms have been recognized implicitly—and often explicitly—by human societies throughout history, and they have been identified by a number of moral philosophers as the ethical prerequisites for personal well-being.[37]

Because these moral norms are assumed to be necessary by those who want to live in a community designed to nurture persons, they are regarded as self-evidently required, that is, as *prima facie* true or valid. It is no wonder, therefore, that important *prima facie* moral obligations such as beneficence, non-maleficence, veracity, justice, and gratitude are accented in codes and discussions of research ethics. For example, the Nuremberg Code and the Declaration of Helsinki emphasize how research on human subjects must benefit society and individual patients, must not harm patients physically and mentally, and must be conducted accurately and truthfully rather than fraudulently or deceitfully.[38(pp 287-293)] These principles are consonant with the emphasis in the Hippocratic Oath, which states that each physician must benefit the sick according to his ability and judgment and keep patients from harm.[38] They also are emphasized in the 1978 Belmont Report Produced by the National Commision for the Protection of Human Subjects of Biomedical and Behavioral Research. This report calls beneficence "an obligation" that includes the principles of not harming patients and of maximizing possible benefits for individual patients and for "members of the larger society."[39] The report also recognizes the importance of the *prima facie* obligations of justice and gratitude. Justice requires that all people be treated equally, that is, that explicit and implicit social, sexual, economic, and age-related biases must not present, as, for example, in recruiting and experimenting on some groups more than others.[39] Gratitude assumes that, as long as research subjects are not harmed, they should feel morally obligated to participate in research out of their indebtedness to society.

It is a mistake to equate *prima facie* ethics with utilitarian ethics. Utilitarianism determines which acts are right or wrong according to a calculation of the greatest pleasure for the greatest number of persons. Utilitarianism thus can be used to justify the harming or sacrificing of one or more individuals for the happiness or pleasure of the majority.[35] Although utilitarianism can be used to justify experimental research without informed consent, this point of view dismisses the importance of the individual.[37,38,40]

In contrast to utilitarianism, which regards the pleasure of the majority as the ultimate good, *prima facie* ethics underlines the necessity of honoring a number of moral goods, each of which must be counterbalanced against one another. Even though this mode of ethical reasoning makes it possible to assume that the individual could express his or her gratitude by contributing to beneficial biomedical research, this perspective requires that this is counterbalanced by the necessity of telling the truth and of not injuring or harming. Individuals are thus protected to a far greater extent by *prima facie* ethics than by utilitarianism.

Respect-for-Person Ethics

Although respect-for-person ethics complements the principles of *prima facie* ethics, it leads to greater protection of the individual. The principle of respect for person is predicated upon the notion that, as persons, human beings are aware that their thoughts, ideas, feelings, reveries, and memories are distinct and separate from those of other persons. It presupposes that, to be a person, one has a sense of biological, cognitive, and emotional privacy[41]; and its moral aim is to enable such persons to exercise control over these realms of privacy. This moral position assumes that persons are sufficiently free to choose different avenues of action and that without this freedom it is nonsensical to blame them for their choices and deeds. In this sense, freedom is a logical prerequisite "for the existence of a moral community."[38,42] Respect-for-person ethics also assumes that each person is the source of respect and value, meaning that he or she can define his or her own ends, rather than be used as a means for the purposes or ends of another. With this respect for the worth and freedom of others, persons can relate to each other out of mutual respect. Without it, relations between persons ultimately are governed by power, force, and violence.

This framework for ethical reasoning is so strongly supported in Anglo-American law that it is appropriately called a "law-like model" of ethical relationships.[43] In contrast to the emphasis on the duties owed to others in *prima facie* ethics, the law—and, behind it, respect-for-person principles—emphasizes that persons are capable of independent action and have the right to think and decide for themselves.[38]

The ethical assumptions of respect for persons also are apparent in most codes and discussions regarding the conduct of moral research. The Nuremberg Code begins with the concept that the "voluntary consent of the human subject is absolutely essential" and stresses that each research subject must be able "to exercise free power of choice, without the intervention of any element of force . . . or coercion."[38] The Declaration of Helsinki asserts that the "integrity" of each research subject must be "respected,"[36] and the Belmont Report lists respect for person as the first of the "basic ethical principles of research."[39]

Respect-for-person ethics requires that each individual must be allowed to consent to or refuse to become involved in research, *whether or not this research is possibly harmful.* Beginning as it does with the autonomy and worth of the individual, this position assumes that the individual has the right to choose when she or he may wish to be benefited, harmed, hassled, or manipulated by others for what may appear to be benign ends.[33] Without this power to choose, human adults become objects that can be used as a means for the ends of others, rather than persons who are active, free agents with the right and power to control how and when they wish to share themselves with others.[44] This serves as a powerful protection to the autonomy and privacy of the individual.

The ethical principles of respect for persons are applied to human research through the obtaining of informed consent. Some medical researchers, however, have discounted or denigrated this requirement. It has been called "no more than an elaborate ritual," easily extracted from subjects by determined investigators,[45] and it sometimes is discounted or dismissed by claims that no subject can be "fully informed" and that truly "free consent" is a myth.[46] The first of these objections is true with respect to what can be and sometimes is done with research subjects, but it is unethical with respect to what should be done with them. The second and third of these objections represent misunderstandings of the fundamental criteria of informed consent, which include *competency, adequate information, comprehension of this information,* and *voluntariness.*

Competency for adults involves their ability to make a decision based on a "reasonable" understanding of the research procedures involved and a weighing of possible harms and benefits. Although dilemmas arise regarding borderline cases of low intelligence, compulsiveness, and mental illness, the principle clearly points to the ability of most persons to choose which course they will follow if the other criteria of informed consent are met. Judgments regarding which subjects are competent or incompetent on the basis of the reasons they give for refusing to consent may mask the value judgments of scientific professionals regarding how rational persons think and to what procedures they will or will not consent.[38] Although judgments concerning competency are by no means cut and dried, they are to be dissociated as much as possible from personal preferences, value orientations, and sectarian or eccentric world views. Definitions of competency are complex and multidimensional and perhaps are defined most accurately and carefully through traditions of law, which tend to be inclusive of diversity and tolerant of broad definitions of rationality.[38]

Research subjects also must be informed. This does not mean that they must be fully informed about all the details and nuances of research; rather, it means that they must be given enough information to make a choice that balances what reasonable persons generally need to know with what each individual person needs to know in order to decide about becoming a subject of research. This information should not be equated with assessments of technical biomedical data made by research professionals or Institutional Review Boards (IRBs).[38-39] Overt or covert deception, of course, is clearly immoral, for it distorts the information required for free choice and represents a using of persons for the ends of the researcher (whether these ends are malicious or well-intentioned), rather than regarding persons as ends in themselves.

The third criterion, comprehension of the information given, is also necessary, for autonomous choice is impossible if the research subject does not comprehend the relevant information pertaining to an experimental protocol. This comprehension is undercut if relevant information is presented in a disorganized fashion and/or is presented too rapidly and/or is not presented on the level of the subject's mental and educational capacities. Difficult ethical dilemmas are raised when patients may wish to waive hearing about and weighing information pertaining to their being entered on research protocols. This is especially significant for cancer patients, because these patients are especially trusting of physician-researchers, are sometimes weak and feel badly, and often have irrelevant or irrational beliefs and expectations regarding the research that is being conducted.

Finally, the fourth criterion, voluntariness, is a requisite for informed consent. The Nuremberg Code expresses this principle strongly: Patients "should be so situated as to be able to exercise free power of choice, without the intervention of any element of force, fraud, deceit, duress, overreaching, or any other ulterior form of constraint or coercion."[38] Coercion occurs when investigators either use some threat of harm in order to obtain compliance or withdraw certain benefits from patients-subjects in order to secure this compliance. "Duress" and "overreaching" are perhaps best called undue influence, and they occur when special rewards or persuasive techniques are used to induce the subjects to comply with the wishes of the researcher against their better judgment.

Ethics and Oncology

There is a certain razor's edge to the discipline of ethics that requires that clear, tough, and limiting judgments be made that hold to the principles that it has arduously clarified over time.[44] We now shall scrutinize important aspects of the value system of clinical oncological research, as seen through the lens of *prima facie* and respect-for-person ethics. This discussion will focus on how a number of the values and value priorities held by many oncologist–researchers would be ordered and shaped by ethics.

Serious value conflicts and worrisome dilemmas are raised when the value system of research in chemotherapy is viewed through *prima facie* and respect-for-person ethics. These conflicts and dilemmas are generated primarily because the values and goods of researchers in chemotherapy tend to override ethical values and goods. This tendency seems so strong that many of the underlying principles of *prima facie* and respect-for-person ethics appear to have a fragile, tenuous status. This is displayed by the following factors, which are intimately and/or inherently linked to some of the fundamental ingredients of research in chemotherapy.

First, the celebrated war on cancer, with its powerful political, economic, and professionally competitive dynamics, as well as its popular news coverage, tempts us to assume that the greater good of the majority outweighs the personal good of those who have forms of cancer that can be investigated. The benefits and rights of cancer patients are by no means dismissed purposefully; they simply appear to be less important than the greater "war," which is assumed to involve the entire society. It is thus very tempting for oncologist–researchers to assume that patient–subjects "owe" something to humankind and the common good.[8]

This greater-good reasoning is an example of utilitarian ethics, by which we can justify easily a dismissal of certain *prima facie* and respect-for-person ethical principles. It may appear that there is a small step between the position that cancer patients *can*, if they wish, contribute something very important to future humanity, and the belief that they *should* be doing so. Yet, with respect to ethics, these are seriously and fundamentally different perspectives. The former respects persons as self-directed, while the latter, "ends-justifies-the-means" reasoning can and does undercut important moral dynamics within *prima facie* ethics and the fundamental notion of individual autonomy within the respect-for-person ethics.*

Second, peer loyalties and pressures can lead easily to a compromising of ethical responsibilities to patient–subjects. Peer pressure to secure high percentages of signups on research protocols and the strong pressure to conduct research in order to advance professionally and to receive academic tenure can function

*References 33, 37–40, 42, 43, 47, 48.

as forces that detract from and sometimes undermine a commitment to the autonomy and equal worth of patients.[8]

Third, the intrinsic dynamics of academic medical centers tend to undercut both *prima facie* and respect-for-person ethical values. Even though the great majority of physicians and other health care professionals hold to high ideals and voice their appreciation of the ethical traditions of medicine, their institutional responsibilities may strain these commitments. Severe time constraints limit communication and personalized care. Schedules that continually rotate staff physicians, residents, and medical students on and off ward service place constraints on continuity of care. And constant pressures, both to keep up with new scientific data in one's medical specialty and to expand the knowledge base of this specialty, can make it difficult, if not impossible, to give maximally beneficial care to patients and relate to them as self-directed individuals.[43]

Fourth, intrinsic to research in oncological chemotherapy is the need to enroll large numbers of research subjects on experimental protocols in order to win incremental battles against cancer. Ethical principles or rules that would curtail or severely restrict the number of research subjects needed for these experiments thus can be viewed as undermining the essential fabric and character of such experiments.

Fifth, the possible psychological needs of oncologist-researchers to compensate for the "loss" of so many patients can make experimental research seem all the more important. Even if these researchers do not view a single experiment as offering significant hope for life prolongation or cure, together these experiments symbolize hope, progress, and a chance to "do something" for patients in dire and heart-rending circumstances.

Sixth, the traditions of cancer care designed to shield patients from possible harms and to benefit them through the maintaining of hope can and do undercut an emphasis on autonomy and rights. The serious dilemmas and conflicts that arise here will be explored in greater detail shortly.

Seventh, given their ardent, sometimes desperate hopes and their great dependence upon and trust in their physician-researchers, patients can be exploited and coerced easily.[8] Vulnerable and extremely suggestible, patient-subjects usually are recruited without difficulty. High percentages of signups thus are achieved readily, once tactical approaches have been carefully developed.

Eighth, many family members also are inclined to pressure their relatives to enroll on research protocols, and they can be co-opted easily to keep "painful" information from these relatives. Although exceptions exist, family members by and large do not represent watchful, critical parties who are knowledgeable of research in chemotherapy. Often, they are not as concerned as they should be about the protection and autonomy of their relatives.

Ninth, as ironic as it may seem, it is unrealistic to assume that IRBs guarantee that research will be conducted ethically. Although IRBs were created initially for the purpose of protecting subjects of research, they in fact perform many roles, some of which devalue this initial mission. For example, the authors of a recent review on the philosophy and purpose of an IRB noted that a general role of their IRB was to "serve the investigator to the best of its ability in reducing paper work and the need for extraneous information."[15:69] Furthermore, even with respect to their reviewing, revising, and approving consent forms, IRBs typically serve several parties. Among other things, consent forms are designed to protect subjects from harm, to avoid fraud, to promote self-scrutiny among medical professionals, to promote rational decisions involving effective research, and to protect the researchers themselves and their respective institutions.[15,38,49] In short, parallel to the several roles assumed by physician-researchers, IRBs perform a number of institutional roles and even utilize consent forms for a number of purposes besides those inherent to research ethics.

The signing of IRB consent forms also does not necessarily assure that the rights of patients are being respected. Ethically and legally, the consent process is based, root and branch, on the actual exchanges between investigator and subject, not on the procuring of signatures. If the investigator so desires, he or she can either highlight the information on consent forms or downplay its importance, the latter either for the purpose of shielding patients from psychological harm or possibly for self-serving ends. It can by no means be assumed that the existence of IRBs generally, and consent forms specifically, guarantees that ethical research is being conducted.

Justifications for Experimentation in Chemotherapy

It is now apparent that a number of the fundamental ingredients of clinical oncological research can conflict with and/or compromise *prima facie* and respect-for-person ethical principles. In fact, it might seem at first that these two value systems are so different that they are intrinsically and theoretically at loggerheads with each other. This, however, does not follow; for it would appear that these ethical modes of reasoning are far more important to research in chemotherapy than the fund-raising justifications some oncologists would suggest.

We have noted how quantitative calculations of dollars spent and returned and "person years" produced have been used for the purpose of securing research funding and conducting further clinical research on human subjects. On the basis of these calculations, oncologists have concluded that chemotherapy has "added immensely" to success rates in cancer treatment.[19] They have noted particularly how approximately 11,000 persons are cured each year and how another 47,500 persons have their lives extended for approximately one year. They also have noted how research in chemotherapy has changed life expectancies dramatically for persons with such malignancies as testicular carcinoma, acute lymphocytic leukemia, and Hodgkin's disease.

Arguments that use quantitative statistics as justifications, however, must be scrutinized carefully. For example, the 11,000 cured represent 4.4 percent of 250,000 inoperable cases of cancer. If we add to this figure the 47,500 patients whose lives are prolonged (plus another 10,000 who might have had some positive response from chemotherapy from this group of 250,000), 21 percent of these inoperable patients experience "some prolongation of survival."[18] Of the approximately 170,000 patients or patient-subjects who are at high risk for a reoccurrence of cancer, 9 percent can benefit from optimal doses of current chemotherapeutic agents.

Not all of the 420,000 patients in both of these populations receive chemotherapy. In fact, it has been estimated that of the approximately 200,000 persons who receive chemotherapeutic drugs each year, the majority (at least 59%) will have to endure varying degrees of nausea, vomiting, ulcerations, hair loss, physical exhaustion, and so on, with little or no benefit.[18] Oncologists have rightly pointed out that these morbidity effects are no more, and are likely less, distressing than the pain and suffering that result if cancer is allowed to run its devastating natural course. But this argument is based significantly on the palliative care that oncologists are able to give. This care also can be given without placing persons on chemotherapy protocols, which likely produce on the whole fewer benefits and greater risks of toxicity and morbidity than standard ones. In short, utilitarian calculations are uncertain warrants for research in chemotherapy.

Granted the weakness of justifying chemotherapy research on the basis of gross mortality and morbidity rates, might it be possible to justify this research on this basis of relative "progress" over time, say, over the last 30 years? While more convincing than gross statistics, this form of reasoning is nevertheless tenuous as a utilitarian argument, that is, as an argument that seeks to justify research on the basis of the greatest amount of good for the greatest number of persons, making use of limited amounts of time and money. For example, the greatest improvements in cancer survival rates occurred in the 1940s and 1950s, before the dramatic upsurge in chemotherapy experimentation happened.[50] In fact, since the advent of heavily funded government programs, survival rate changes with chemotherapeutic agents have been relatively limited.[18] While survival rates for some tumors like testicular carcinoma or acute lymphocytic leukemia in children are dramatic, between 1940 and 1970 survival rates increased incrementally for most types of neoplasms: approximately 15 percent for colon and rectal cancers, 9 percent for breast cancers, and 20 percent for cancer of the larynx. Mortality rates remained at 2 percent for pancreatic malignancies.[50] Furthermore, the great reliance at the present time on combination therapy indicates that most experiments with anticancer drugs are calculated to discover incremental changes in mortality rates, not quantitative leaps or stunning breakthroughs. Quantitative measurements of progress over time thus are limited in their convincingness, even though such calculations constantly permeate the thought of many oncologist-researchers.

Rather than relying on utilitarian calculations, it would appear that the best moral arguments for this research and experimentation are linked to the great, perhaps inestimable value of the individual—the 4.4 percent who are cured, rather than the majority who are slightly or negligibly affected. Given the consummate value of individual persons, it makes sense to have spent great effort, time, and money over the course of 30 years to be able to prolong the lives of 9 percent or 15 percent to 20 percent of patients and patient-subjects with specific forms of malignant neoplasms. In actuality, this person-centered orientation is implicit and powerful within the practice of oncology. Indeed, quantitative calculations of cure and life-prolongation rates seem to detract from the fundamental character of this subspecialty, which has focused over time on curing a relatively small number of persons in the face of toxicity and pain. Sensing this, some chemotherapists point out that they cannot justify their professional interventions morally by mortality rates alone. Instead, they vindicate their efforts morally by believing that personally and psychologically they benefit individual patients who come in search of cure, or relief, or solace.

The ethical theories that focus precisely on the value of persons are *prima facie* and respect-for-person ethics. Oncologist-researchers thus can be consistent logically and morally if they utilize the principles from these ethical traditions both to justify fully the worth of their research and to relate to those who become—or might become—subjects of research.

Harms and Benefits

In order to govern their medical interventions by certain principles from *prima facie* ethics, principles that are in keeping with the Hippocratic tradition, it is necessary that physicians perform treatments that are more likely to benefit than to harm patients. Given the fact that cancer is an extreme illness, physicians uphold this moral perspective when they administer extreme treatments, as long as these treatments are more likely to benefit than to harm patients.[39] Whether this principle can be used to justify Phase I cancer experimentation, however, is an open question, because there is so much disagreement over whether these studies offer more benefit than harm to patient-subjects.

Some oncologists seriously question whether potential benefits can ever outweigh possible harms in Phase I trials, because these experiments are designed primarily to produce, measure, and define toxicity effects, not to determine which cancers will respond most significantly to which drugs.[8] Furthermore, potential benefits are greatly limited at the beginning of Phase I studies, when impotent doses are being administered to avoid unknown toxic effects. In the meantime, the risks of toxicity and mortality are greatest in Phase I trials, when the actions of experimental drugs or drug combinations are understood only partially from prior animal trials.[51]

Other physicians claim that all phases of cancer research, including Phase I studies, are moral because oncological drugs are tested with a "therapeutic intent" and each phase represents "the optimal type of care that a patient with a disease not easily amenable to treatment can receive."[13] It also has been claimed that Phase I studies "sometimes result in significant responses."[1]

In scrutinizing these positions ethically, it would appear that "therapeutic intent" hardly constitutes "benefit," and the "significant responses" that have been claimed for some Phase I studies in any case should be specified and proven in order for them to bear weight. This points to a general need: Serious and open discussions should be conducted in order to clear up the uncertainties and disagreements that exist over the possible benefits and harms of Phase I studies.

"The optimal type of care" that subjects may receive in Phase I studies also needs to be clarified. If this refers to anticancer therapeutic response, then "optimal" must be spelled out in terms of statistical possibilities or probabilities. Compared to a zero response rate, a 10,000-to-one chance of an anticancer response might be called "optimal," but it is questionable whether this constitutes more "benefit" than harm. On the other hand, if "optimal care" is a shorthand phrase for the tradition of using experimental drugs in order to fend off the patient–subjects' feelings of helplessness and to maintain hope, other ethical questions are raised. In this instance, somewhat debatable psychological benefits are being offered to patient–subjects, while clear professional benefits are gained by some researchers—especially those who coordinate research efforts. This raises serious questions over conflicting loyalties and mixed motives. Furthermore, the stated and public purpose of chemotherapy research is the discovery of better cancer cures, rather than a treating of the psychological and emotional states of patients or patient–subjects per se. If, indeed, much experimental research serves primarily as a substitute for psychotherapy, this needs to be stated publicly, empirically validated, and utilized in informed consents. These issues and dilemmas do not necessarily mean that it is impossible to use harm-benefit analysis to justify Phase I research. They do, however, call into question a number of the attempts that have been made thus far to harness this tradition of ethical reasoning in order to justify these trials.

Truth-Telling

Truth-telling, or veracity, is a fundamental moral principle, both within *prima facie* and respect-for-person ethics. Within the latter tradition truthful information is essential for informed consent and personal autonomy. Within the former, truth-telling is one of several right-making moral duties that at times can be overruled by the more stringent duties of beneficence and nonmalfeasance. For example, lying is morally permissible (although still not virtuous) in the classic instance of replying to the Gestapo, during World War II, if asked whether one is harboring a Jewish family. Here veracity is set aside for the more stringent moral obligation of protecting other persons from torture or death.

Parallel to *prima facie* moral reasoning, medical practitioners have on occasion regarded truthfulness to patients as secondary to their being harmed or benefited. Cancer specialists, for example, have in the past advocated outright deception if this protects patients from psychological harm,[52] and at other times they have sought to limit how much truth is told in order to shield patients from undue trauma.[9,53] Might it therefore be morally acceptable for oncologist–researchers to keep part of the "painful truth" from research subjects in order either to benefit them by maintaining hope[7] or to protect them from acute anxiety or depression?[9] This would appear to conform not only with the reluctance-to-tell tradition within cancer care but also with *prima facie* moral reasoning.

This shielding of patients from truthful information, however, presents problems that also seem out of harmony with *prima facie* ethics. First, if it actually were true that accurate information concerning the patient's diagnosis and/or prognosis often would lead to suicide attempts, psychotic breakdowns, and severe depression (as was once thought), it would be morally permissible to keep accurate information from patients and at times to tell falsehoods.[52] But psychological studies of grief and loss during the last 30 years have called into question these traditional intuitions. Shock and grief now are understood as predictable, patterned, manageable "syndromes," which, although painful and trying, are not marked by frequent, devastating, traumatic harms. Although it is true that many patients suffer "acute anxiety" when cancer diagnosis is confirmed or when they discover that they have failed to respond to treatment,[54] contemporary research on grief and loss indicates that shock and initial disorientation represent a reactive "stage," which is followed by a recovering of one's bearings and abilities to understand, assess, and decide what one wishes to do.[47,54] It appears to be false—and also possibly self-serving—to assume that patients remain so confused and traumatized that they cannot make decisions about their future or give informed consent.[55] Furthermore, it seems that much of the anxiety, sense of loss, and depression experienced by patients can be significantly or greatly alleviated with the aid and support of the caring and knowledgeable physician.[54]

Second, contrary to the reluctance-to-tell tradition within cancer care, current writers emphasize that more psychological harm than benefit occurs when patients are not informed. One study has indicated that a lack of forthright information contributes to long-term emotional upsets.[54] It even appears that, when patients in consultation with their physicians are granted a choice regarding the treatments they may want to follow, their psychological difficulties will be minimized.[54,56] In short, forthrightness and truthfulness appear to benefit cancer patients far more than silence and/or deception.

Special problems related to truth-telling also are raised over other aspects of chemotherapy experimentation. First, it seems to be relatively common for experimental drugs to be recommended for human patients because these drugs "have shown promise in animal studies." Although true in itself, this statement can be highly misleading unless the patient is informed of the discrepancies between response rates in animals and the likely response rates in humans.[3,8] Without such clarifications, prospective subjects of research are deceived easily by false hopes. Although statements to the effect that physician–researchers "simply do not know" about human response rates are more accurate than statistics about promising cures, what is known or not known still needs some kind of operational or "confidence level" definition.[51]

Second, and closely related to the first, after chemotherapists have shared negative news with patients, they may respond to the effect that, "We still have drugs that we are excited about. . . ." Such statements, if explained, can be truthful and realistic; but, if left unexplained, they can be, and likely are, deceiving. They mask the truth if the investigator has in mind the limited, but nevertheless important, incremental statistical cures and life-prolongation rates of drug combination experiments, while the research subject quite naturally has in mind a radically different set of expectations. He or she may well interpret these statements in terms of promising images of Interferon on magazine covers, of other unrelated technological breakthroughs, or general impressions of highly promising cures in the armamentarium of modern medicine. The principle of veracity calls for a forthright, common-sense bridging of these vastly different messages.

Finally, it is the responsibility of IRBs to require that consent forms truthfully and completely outline the probable benefits and risks of all phases of biomedical research. Some IRBs require statements like the following: "I understand that this treatment may not do me any good, and in fact may make me worse." Although this language points out the likely harms of Phase I or Phase II studies, it nevertheless can create false expectations. While aware that these experiments are possibly ineffective and/or harmful, research subjects can believe easily that their chances for benefit and care are far greater than truthful data would indicate. This is all the more probable if investigators interpret IRB consent forms enthusiastically and optimistically.

Autonomous Persons

Up to this point I have been dealing primarily with the way certain *prima facie* ethical principles raise worrisome ethical dilemmas regarding the conducting and justifying of chemotherapy research. An equally, if not more, problematic "fit" exists, however, between some of the operating principles of adult oncological experimentation and respect-for-person ethical principles. Respect-for-person ethics requires that persons are respected as autonomous, free agents who are allowed to choose their own courses of action. Yet, as we have noted, many of the ingredients of oncological research tend to undercut or seriously devalue the autonomy or self-direction of the individual.

As tenuous and frail as it may be within the value system of clinical oncological research, the autonomy of the individual is all the more important if persons are to have control over their cognitive, physical, emotional, and spiritual integrity. Professionals in law, religion, psychology, and medicine are trained to recognize and make decisions concerning what counts for harms, injuries, and benefits. These decisions easily are taken to mean that highly trained professionals are to make decisions *for* their clients, patients, or subjects, rather than to make professional judgments that these persons then are allowed to accept or possibly alter or reject. Unless the individual person is granted the right to decide what counts for her or his own harms or benefits, she or he easily can be manipulated by others rather than function as a self-willed person who defines her or his own ends.

These issues engender serious problems in anticancer experimentation. Within the subdiscipline of oncology, for example, "radical amputations or major alterations of normal organs and to their functions" are considered "acceptable forms" of treatment, even if the individual who is treated "never returns to normal" life and has to live with "residual injury."[55] Given the lethal or life-threatening nature of malignant neoplasms, these alternatives make sense to numerous patients, as well as to the oncologists who specialize in cancer treatment. Yet, who is to decide when these treatments will be utilized? Respect-for-person ethics emphasize that each individual person must be granted the right to make his or her own informed choices with respect to such treatments. These therapies may be "acceptable," but they also must be chosen or accepted. This is critically important in chemotherapy experimentation and also must be seriously considered within the general practice of oncology.

With respect to who defines what counts as harms or benefits, consider morbidity. Are the degrees of nausea, vomiting, ulcerations, and risks of organ damage to be assessed as "temporary, predictable, and manageable,"[1] or are they "ugly and violent"?[3,4] Is hair loss a bothersome side-effect because it reminds patients and family that someone has cancer,[19] or is it a source of embarrassment and possible shame that is to be hidden from friends, yet willingly endured for the sake of ultimate cure?[25] These assessments and reactions vary with those who are doing the evaluating, and the principle of autonomy within respect-for-person ethics emphasizes that those who are affected must be able to exercise ultimate choice over what they will or will not endure.

This principle of free choice does not mean that prospective subjects of research will always or even frequently refuse to enroll on research protocols and endure these treatments in the light of what they will face if their disease runs its "natural course." As free to choose, these persons can and should be allowed to try "long shots" for the sake of cure. They can, and likely will, choose morbidity as a result of clinical research over possible, probable, or certain mortality. They also may choose to become subjects of research in order to contribute to the common good or display gratitude out of a sense of moral duty. Respect for persons simply means that in all cases they should be free to choose.

As noted previously, the autonomy of the individual is secured in research through informed consent, and informed consent involves competency, truthful information, a comprehension of this information, and voluntariness. The preceding discussion of truth-telling points to some of the dilemmas associated with giving correct information to research subjects. In order for persons to be autonomous, this information must be presented clearly, accurately, and in common-sense terms and must be detailed enough for "reasonable persons" to make choices. The essential information called for includes the following: the purpose(s), risks, and anticipated benefits of the research; its procedures; the right to withdraw at any time from the research protocol; the opportunity to ask questions; the costs, length, time, and number of interventions required by the research; and, for research on therapeutic procedures or agents, a discussion of alternative procedures.[38,39] The most crucial information deals with the purposes, risks, and anticipated benefits of the research. Effective, time-efficient ways of communicating this information can be developed and practiced.

Concerning comprehension, intellectual and psychological biases can consciously or unconsciously influence what professionals believe ordinary persons can understand. Some writers have urged, for example, that cancer patients "ought to be given only as much as they are intellectually able to comprehend" and " emotionally able to integrate."[54] This easily serves as a rationale for keeping important information from patients rather than as a challenge to see that essential information is clearly and deliberately communicated in simple language. The principle of autonomy necessitates effective communication. Skill in communication is thus a moral prerequisite for those who secure the informed consent of research subjects. One of the most effective measurements of how much has been comprehended involves the investigator's having each research subject express in his or her own words what has been communicated.[53]

Finally, informed consent—and, behind it, respect-for-person ethics—requires that research subjects should volunteer or "fully consent" to becoming enrolled on research protocols. Sensitive, serious, and possibly insolvable problems are raised by this principle; for, on the one hand, as psychologically vulnerable and suggestible, cancer patients easily are coerced and pressured to sign up for research experiments. On the other hand, the ingredients of oncological research in the academic teaching hospital presuppose that these experiments are immensely valuable. The complex, sensitive, and open-ended questions raised by these circumstances need to be carefully, critically, and openly discussed.

As noted previously, the principle of voluntariness required that prospective research subjects are neither coerced nor unduly influenced. This means that certain actions must be avoided by chemotherapy researchers if subjects are respected as autonomous persons. It is coercive, for example, for investigators either to imply or state outright that if patients become enrolled on research protocols, they will receive better care; if they sign up, they will be monitored with particular care, given the latest and best pain medication, and incorporated into an active, working "team" of physician–researchers and other medical professionals; while, if they do not consent to become research subjects, they will receive less expert and personalized care. They will, for example, become the patients of medical residents, or perhaps be dismissed from the hospital, with the implication that their pain and sickness will not be monitored. These approaches to prospective subjects of chemotherapy research have been called "brutally coercive," and rightly viewed as contradictory to the Hippocratic tradition of caring for and benefiting all patients.[8] According to respect-for-person ethical principles as well, these actions are indeed coercive.

One of the most poignant problems of cancer care in academic medical centers is raised by these actions taken toward patients, because these actions realistically reflect some of the dynamics of the teaching, research-oriented hospital. The institutions in which the researching physician works are designed to utilize the time and efforts of full-time teaching and researching physicians "efficiently." Their roles are defined so that they can focus on complicated cases and clinical research, and curative rather than palliative care is accented. Meanwhile, residents and medical students are expected to develop an initial knowledge of disease diagnosis and treatment and learn how to deliver care to many types of patients, including cancer patients. In short, the dynamics of the teaching hospital make it extremely difficult for staff physicians not to be "coercive" in terms of the levels of care that will or will not be received by patients if they do or do not become enrolled on experimental protocols. To imply that the cancer patients who refuse to become enrolled will receive the same levels of expert care as those who do consent simply may not be true.

It would seem, therefore, that many, if not most, chemotherapy researchers function within an ipso facto coercive environment. If they wish to do clinical research, they must accept the time constraints and teaching and training mandates of the institution where this research is being conducted. Regardless of good will and ethical sensitivity, certain of their actions toward prospective research subjects likely will constitute coercive levels of pressure. This means, that if ethical principles of respect for persons are to be honored, institutional procedures and policies must be reviewed and redesigned.

Finally, the principle of autonomy does not require that physician-researchers accent only the negative effects and risks of chemotherapy treatments or avoid trying to convince research subjects that a given protocol may be beneficial. To the contrary, informed consent calls for a full display of benefits as well as harms. Most chemotherapy researchers rightly and realistically know what the effects of untreated cancer are on the human body, mind, and spirit.

It is thus important for them to describe the prognosis of untreated cancer along with the prognosis of experimental therapy. It is probably impossible to draw a clear line between unjustifiable pressure and warranted influence with respect to the possible benefits and harms of experimental procedures, as weighed against the competing wants, needs, and family interests of prospective subjects of research. The ethical traditions utilized in this essay would put the matter in these terms: Prospective research subjects are to be respected as self-directed persons who are allowed to make their own choices after justifiable, noncoercive attempts at persuasion by investigators are completed.

Conclusion

Incorporated as they are within the dynamics of their subspecialties, chemotherapy researchers themselves ultimately are responsible for the ways patients and prospective research subjects are related to ethically. IRBs are commissioned to monitor certain of these relationships, but, as we have noted, IRBs are limited in influence and sometimes are resisted and stereotyped as intrusive and bureaucratic. It is hoped that this essay will encourage oncologist–researchers to further assess and clarify their moral and nonmoral values and priorities and to address forthrightly the issues outlined here. The shaping of biomedical interventions according to the ordinary principles of human morality is in accord with the nature and purpose of medical ethics.

References

1. DeVita VT: DeVita's response to *Post* article. *The Washington Post,* Monday, October 19, 1981, A27.
2. Gray BH, Cooke RA, Tannenbaum AS: Research involving human subjects. *Science* 201:1094–1101, 1978.
3. Gup T, Neumann, J: Experimental drugs: Death in the search for cures. *The Washington Post,* Sunday, October 18, 1981, A1, A14–15.
4. Gup T, Neumann, J: Risk, rivalry and research—and error. *The Washington Post,* Monday, October 19, 1981, A26–27.
5. Gup T, Neumann, J: The world of shattered hopes. *The Washington Post,* Tuesday, October 20, 1981, A1, A18–19.
6. Gup T, Neumann J: Spark of hope versus ordeal of pain: Dilemma of drug researchers. *The Washington Post,* Wednesday, October 21, 1981, A1, A10.
7. Leventhal BG: Letter to Jonathan Neumann, Monday, October 12, 1981.
8. Krant MJ, Cohen JL, Rosenbaum C: Moral dilemmas in clinical cancer experimentation. *Med Pediatr Oncol* 3:141–147, 1977.
9. Shingleton WW, Shingleton AB: Ethical considerations in the treatment of breast cancer. *Cancer* 46:1031–1034, 1980.

10. Blanchard CG, Ruckdeschel JC, Cohen RE, et al: Attitudes toward cancer. *Cancer* 47:2756–2762, 1981.
11. Neidhart JA, Gagen M, Young D, et al: Specific antiemetics for specific cancer chemotherapeutic agents. *Cancer* 47:1439–1443, 1981.
12. Reed ML, Vait Kevicius VK, Al-Sarraf M, et al: The practicality of chronic hepatic artery infusion therapy of primary and metastatic hepatic malignancies. *Cancer* 47:402–409, 1981.
13. Muggia FM, DeVita VT: Letter to the editor, *Med Pediatr Oncol* 4:181, 1978.
14. Higgins GA: Problems in clinical trials: Lessons from the 'tuck uppers.' *Cancer* 47:2167–2171, 1981.
15. Brown JHU, Schoenfeld L, Allan PW: The philosophy of an institutional review board for the protection of human subjects. *J M Educ* 55:67–69, 1980.
16. Millman M: *The Unkindest Cut.* New York, Morrow Quill Paperbacks, 1977.
17. Silverberg E: Cancer statistics, 1982. *CA* 32:15–31, 1982.
18. DeVita VT Jr, Henney JE, Hubbard SM: Estimation of the numerical and economic impact of chemotherapy in the treatment of cancer, in Burchenal JH, Oettgen HF (eds): *Cancer.* New York, Grune and Stratten, 1981, vol 2.
19. Cadman E: Toxicity of chemotherapeutic agents, in Becker FF (ed): *Cancer: A Comprehensive Treatise.* New York, Plenum Press, 1977, vol 5, pp 59–111.
20. Apple MA: New anticancer drug design: Past and present strategies, in Becker FF (ed): *Cancer: A Comprehensive Treatise.* New York, Plenum Press, 1977, pp 599–652.
21. Kaplan BS, Gault MH, Kraak J: Nephropathy as a consequence of neoplasms or their treatment, in Klastersky J, Staquet MJ (eds): *Medical Complications in Cancer Patients.* New York, Raven Press, 1981, pp 135–153.
22. Rozensweig M, Piccart M, Van Hoff PD: Cardiac disorders in cancer patients, in Klastersky J, Staquet MJ (eds): *Medical Complications in Cancer Patients.* New York, Raven Press, 1981, pp 211–230.
23. Von Hoff DD, Pollard E: Gastrointestinal complications of neoplasms, in Klastersky J, Staquet MJ (eds): *Medical Complications in Cancer Patients.* New York, Raven Press, 1981, pp 205–210.
24. Bonica JJ: Cancer pain, in Klastersky J, Staquet MJ (eds): *Medical Complications in Cancer Patients.* New York, Raven Press, 1981, pp 87–115.
25. Fiore N: Fighting cancer—one patient's perspective, *New Engl J of Med* 300:284–289, 1979.
26. Klastersky J, DeJager R: Cutaneous complications in cancer patients, in Klastersky J, Staquet MJ (eds): *Medical Complications in Cancer Patients.* New York, Raven Press, 1981, pp 187–203.
27. Muggia FM, Wilson JK, Weiss RB: Respiratory complications during cancer therapy: Diagnosis and management, in Klastersky J, Staquet MJ (eds): *Medical Complications in Cancer Patients.* New York, Raven Press, 1981, pp 171–186.

28. Veatch HM: Medical ethics: Professional or universal? *Harvard Theol Rev* 65:531-559, 1972.
29. Clark RL: The impact of the national cancer program, in Burchenal JH, Oettgen HF (eds), *Cancer*. New York, Grune and Stratten, 1981, vol 2.
30. Big IF in Cancer. *Time,* March 31, 1980, 60–66.
31. Cabot R: Medical ethics in the hospital. *Nosokomeion*: 151–161, 1931.
32. Levine RJ: Clarifying the concepts of research ethics. *The Hastings Cent Rep,* June 1979, 21–26.
33. Veatch RA: The national commission on IRBs: An evolutionary approach. *Hastings Cent Rep,* February 1979, 22–28.
34. Ingelfinger FJ: The unethical in medical ethics. *Ann Intern Med* 83:264–269, 1975.
35. Fletcher J: Ethical considerations in biomedical research involving human beings. *Bull WHO* 55:101–110, 1977.
36. Clouser KD: Some things medical ethics is not. *JAMA* 223:787–789, 1973.
37. Dyck AJ: *On Human Care.* Nashville, Abingdon Press, 1977.
38. Beauchamp TL, Childress JF: *Principles of Biomedical Ethics.* New York, Oxford University Press, 1979, pp 289–293.
39. The National Commission for the Protection of Human Subjects of Biomedical and Behavioral Research, *Belmont Report.* Washington, DC, DHEW, Publication #78-0012, 1978.
40. Vanderpool HY: B.F. Skinner on ethics on the control of retarded persons. *The Linacre Quarterly* 45:135–151, 1978.
41. Reiman JH: Privacy, intimacy, and personhood. *Phil and Pub Affairs* 6:33–44, 1976.
42. Engelhardt HT Jr: Basic ethical principles in the conduct of biomedical and behavioral research involving human subjects. *Tex Rep Bio Med* 38:139–169, 1979.
43. Erde EL, Vanderpool HY: *The Sources and Character of Medical Values and Medical Ethics.* Galveston, Tex, University of Texas Medical Branch, 1981.
44. Ramsey P: The ethics of a cottage industry in an age of community and research medicine. *New Engl J of Med* 284:700–706, 1971.
45. Ingelfinger FJ: Informed (but uneducated) consent. *New Engl J of Med* 287:466, 1972.
46. Lacher MJ: Patients and physicians as obstacles to a randomized trial. *Semin in Oncol* 8:424–429, 1981.
47. Vanderpool HY: The responsibilities of physicians towards dying patients, in Klastersky J, Staquet MJ (eds): *Medical Complications in Cancer Patients.* New York, Raven Press, 1981, pp 117–134.
48. Veatch RM: Why get consent? *Hosp Physician,* December 1975, 30–31.
49. Smith HL: Ethical consideration in research involving human subjects. *Ethics Sci Med* 6:167–175, 1979.
50. Levin DL, Devesa SS, et al: *Cancer Rates and Risks,* ed 2. Bethesda, National Cancer Institute, DHEW, 1974.
51. Wikler D: Ethical considerations in randomized clinical trials. *Semin Oncol* 8:437–441, 1981.

52. Kline NS, Sobin J: The psychological management of cancer cases. *JAMA* 146:1547–1551, 1951.
53. Holland JF, Frei E III: Principles of management, in Holland JF (ed): *Cancer Medicine*. Philadelphia, Lea and Febiger, 1973, pp 489–498.
54. Krant MJ: Psychological aspects of cancer diagnosis, in Klastersky J, Staquet MJ (eds): *Medical Complications in Cancer Patients*. New York, Raven Press, 1981, pp 69–86.
55. Hackett TP: Psychological assistance for the dying patient and his family. *Ann Rev Med* 27:371–378, 1976.
56. Schain WS: Patients' rights in decision making: the case for personalism versus paternalism in health care. *Cancer* 46:1031–1034, 1980.

Bibliography

Brantner, John. Life-threatening disease as a manageable crisis. *Seminars in Oncology*, June 1974, 153–157.

DeVita, Vincent T. Letter to the editor, *The Washington Post*, October 21, 1981.

Herbert, Victor. Informed consent—a legal evaluation. *Cancer*, 46, 1980, 1042–1044.

Hill Hearings on Cancer Drugs Planned. *The Washington Post*, October 21, 1981, A24.

Ihde, Daniel C., Cohen, Martin, Simms, E., et al. Evaluation of response to chemotherapy with fiberoptic bronchoscopy in non-small cell lung cancer. *Cancer*, 45, 1980, 1693–1696.

Meyerowitz, Beth E., Sparks, F., Spears, I. Adjuvant chemotherapy for breast carcinoma. *Cancer*, 43, 1979, 1613–1618.

Morris, John McLean. Risk/benefit ratios in the management of gynecologic cancer. *Cancer*, 48, 1981, 642–649.

Muss, Human B., et al. Written informed consent in patients with breast cancer. *Cancer*, 43, 1979, 1549–1556.

Neumann, Jonathan. A long, hit-and-miss war against cancer. *The Washington Post*, October 18, 1981, A16.

Ramsey, Paul. *The Patient is Person*. New Haven: Yale University Press, 1970.

Ratzan, Richard M. "Being old makes you different": The ethics of research with elderly subjects. *The Hastings Center Report*, October 1980, 32–42.

Robertson, John A. Legal considerations in clinical cancer research. *Seminars in Oncology*, 8, Fall 1976, 33–44.

Simmons, Paul D. The "human" as a problem in bioethics. *Review and Expositor*, 78, Winter 1981, 91–108.

Sutherland, Arthur M. Psychological impact of cancer and its therapy. *Ca—A Cancer Journal for Clinicians*, 31, May/June 1981, 159–171.

Van Melsen, A.G.M. Person. *Encyclopedia of Bioethics*, vol. 3. New York: The Free Press, 1978, pp 1206–1210.

Vanderpool, Harold Y. The ethics of terminal care. *Journal of the American Medical Association*, 239, February 1978, 850–852.

3

Information Resources for Improved Communication among Cancer Researchers and Clinicians*

Hortencia M. Hornbeak, John H. Schneider, and Dianne E. Tingley

Introduction

The rapidly expanding cancer research effort over the last 10 years has resulted in a logarithmic growth of information. Results of cancer research are published in more than 3,000 biomedical journals and presented at hundreds of scientific conferences each year. It has become increasingly difficult, if not impossible, for investigators to keep abreast of this massive amount of widely dispersed information.

In an effort to respond to specific needs of cancer scientists, several organizations in various countries around the world have developed cancer information resources. A *Directory of Cancer Research Information Resources*[1] provides a comprehensive list of the types of resources available worldwide, along with a detailed description of each service and a contact person. (See Table 3-1 for a list of the types of resources covered in the directory.) This chapter, however, will focus primarily on the technical information services of the National Cancer Institute.

In recognition of the need to collect and disseminate systematically

Table 3-1

Areas Covered in the *Directory of Cancer Research Information Resources*

Computer-based information systems and services
    Databases
    Search centers and services
    Information centers and programs
Primary publications
Secondary publications
Research projects information sources
    Publications
    Data collection centers and organizations
    Databases
Cancer organizations, societies, centers, and funding agencies listed by country
    (excluding U.S. Government agencies)
U.S. Government agencies, products and services
Dial-access services (primarily for health professionals)
Libraries (listed by country with emphasis on cancer-related publications)
Selected classification schemes
    Classification of neoplastic diseases and tumors and clinical procedures
    Classification of cancer research subject areas
Special collections
    Pathology specimens and slides
    Sources of research materials
    Special data collections
Audiovisual information sources

---

information resulting from cancer research, the U.S. Congress mandated in the National Cancer Act of 1971 (Public Law 92-218) that the NCI shall:

> Collect, analyze, and disseminate all data useful in the prevention, diagnosis and treatment of cancer, including the establishment of an international cancer research data bank to collect, catalog, store and disseminate insofar as feasible the results of cancer research undertaken in any country for the use of any person involved in cancer research in any country.

In response to this mandate, the International Cancer Research Data Base (ICRDB) Program of the National Cancer Institute was established in 1974 to provide a comprehensive range of technical information services. The ICRDB Program is unique in that data are collected at every stage of the research process: at the time of funding, as soon as the earliest results of a research effort are presented at a professional meeting or special conference, when a formal article is published, and when books or reviews discuss the research results. In addition, a complete abstract or annotation is provided with each citation.

    This approach is designed to provide information to researchers during the years that often elapse between the initial funding of a research project or activation of a cancer therapy protocol, and the formal publication of results in a scientific journal. By closing this gap, the ICRDB Program hopes to foster better and more timely communication among investigators working in similar research areas at the earliest stages of a project, avoid unnecessary duplication of effort, increase investigators' awareness of new developments in their areas of interest, and promote rapid transfer of applicable research results to the research clinicians.

To accomplish this timely information transfer, the ICRDB Program fully utilizes modern information science technology for the collection, printing, and dissemination of information. Abstracts of articles or scientific presentations and summaries of protocols are prepared by specialists who type the first draft of the abstract at computer terminals. This input is converted to computer files called databases and made available online, which means the data resides permanently in the memory of a central computer. Users at remote locations can search the database, usually through use of terminals connected to the central computer by telephone lines. Researchers can obtain a printout of any desired subset of the information by using a "search profile" to retrieve specific abstracts.

In addition to the databases, the ICRDB Program produces a number of publications that are designed to provide data to basic and clinical researchers in a highly targeted and selective fashion. The publications are prepared by subject specialists who carefully select, analyze, and organize abstracts into a comprehensive spectrum of cancer research areas. The input from specialists ensures that each issue of an ICRDB publication deals in a logical fashion with a specific aspect of cancer information that is most likely to meet the information needs of a targeted group of cancer researchers. The resulting publications, with trivial and marginal material eliminated, provide a focused and convenient source of the latest information on specific topics. Cancer researchers can use these publications to locate specific subsets of information that provide ideas for new or modified areas of research. The publications produced by the ICRDB Program provide information that scientists do not find by scanning a few journals or going to occasional meetings.

As shown in Figure 3-1, the ICRDB Program collects and disseminates three major types of cancer-related information on all aspects of cancer research: clinical protocol summaries, cancer research project descriptions, and abstracts of published literature. The data are stored in three separate databases. Before inclusion in a database, each record is indexed to facilitate retrieval. Every effort is made to ensure that the collected data accurately represent research activity worldwide and are processed quickly so that they can be available to researchers on a timely basis. Figure 3-1 also shows how the collected data are incorporated into technical documents that are disseminated directly to cancer researchers and clinicians.

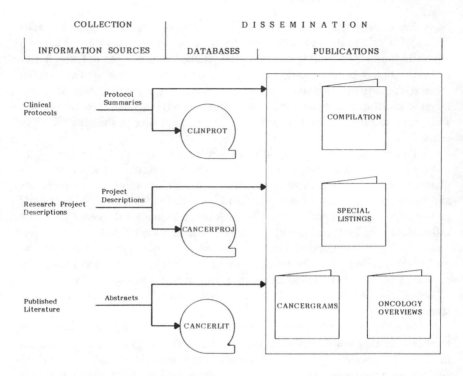

Figure 3-1. Flow Chart of Major ICRDB Products and Services

　　　　In the following discussion of this comprehensive model system, developed by the ICRDB Program, emphasis will be placed on (1) the technical information products and services that maximize the worldwide availability of the collected information and (2) special projects that encourage the international exchange of information by scientists from various countries.

ICRDB Online Databases

Cancer information is collected through a worldwide network of investigators and organizations. This information is used to build and update three databases, collectively known as CANCERLINE. Cancer researchers throughout the world have easy access to this useful and growing store of archival cancer information through a large biomedical information network called MEDLARS (Medical Literature Analysis and Retrieval System), which is operated by the National Library of Medicine and linked to terminals at more than 2,000 locations connected to MEDLARS centers in 14 countries around the world. As of

1981, CANCERLINE became easily available to cancer researchers throughout Europe via a new communication system called EURONET, which is linked to centers that provide CANCERLINE database services in England and Germany.

The three databases (see Figure 3-1) are CLINPROT which contains clinical protocol information; CANCERPROJ, which contains descriptions of current cancer projects; and CANCERLIT, which contains abstracts of the published cancer literature. The CLINPROT and CANCERPROJ databases are updated quarterly, and the CANCERLIT database is updated monthly.

The CLINPROT database contains over 2,900 summaries of experimental clinical protocol trials carried out at centers in the United States, Europe, and other countries over the past six years. More than 1,500 of these protocols are still open to patient entry. Cancer therapy protocols for the CLINPROT database are throughout the world. Summaries of each protocol are prepared by subject specialists and returned to the group chairperson or the principal investigator for final review to ensure the accuracy of the summarized data. Currency is achieved by collecting updated information and using it to revise each protocol on a regular basis. All protocols are indexed by tumor site and specific therapeutic agent or combination of agents. Protocol summaries can be retrieved from the database by using a simple search profile. Each summary describes the objectives of the protocol, the entry criteria, an outline of the arms of the study, the agents used, the dosage schedules, the stratification criteria, and patient accrual data. This information is useful to clinicians who are designing new clinical trials or who wish to refer patients to open protocols.

The CANCERPROJ database contains some 21,000 descriptions of current cancer research projects, 5,000 of which are received from 85 countries outside the United States through an ICRDB-supported Current Cancer Research Project Analysis Center. Through the combined efforts of this center, the staff of the International Union Against Cancer (UICC) located in Geneva, Switzerland, and data coordinators in many countries, the ICRDB Program has received cancer-related project descriptions from funding organizations and from principal investigators throughout the world.

Project descriptions include project title, author, address, and a summary of the objectives, approach, and results to date. Prior to the establishment of this database, much of the information on cancer research activities in other countries was widely scattered or unavailable. Now, investigators around the world can retrieve information on research projects in their specific areas of interest by a simple search of CANCERPROJ. The availability of this type of information promotes collaboration and facilitates cooperation among researchers working in similar areas of cancer research.

The CANCERLIT database is a useful and comprehensive archival source of information on the results of cancer research that have been published over the past two decades. It now contains nearly 300,000 English-language abstracts of articles from scientific journals, papers presented at scientific meetings, books, theses, government reports, and other monographs. Some 3,000 different scientific journals are screened on a regular basis by subject specialists to identify articles dealing with cancer. Author abstracts are used when publisher permission for such use has been granted. For other articles, abstracts are prepared by subject specialists. The inclusion of some 8,000 to 10,000 abstracts of cancer-related papers presented at scientific meetings each year is particularly useful because these abstracts often describe very recent results that would not be available as a formal publication for many months, if not a year or more. To our knowledge, no other cancer information service provides this type of timely and useful information.

About 40,000 new abstracts are added to the CANCERLIT database each year. Since abstracts are prepared within 30 days after receipt of a publication, and since the database is updated monthly, scientists have convenient and rapid access to current information within two months after it is published. Emphasis has been placed on providing abstracts of all articles, since the abstracts can be used, in most cases, to determine whether an article is sufficiently relevant or substantive to justify reading the complete article. Often, the abstract alone provides enough information to avoid the time and effort needed to locate the article. In contrast, many other information services provide only titles and citations or a limited number of abstracts, thereby requiring the user to locate the article to determine its usefulness.

Abstracts are retrieved by online searching using any word or combination of words that appears in the title or text of the abstracts. If only a few abstracts are retrieved or the need for them is urgent, they can be displayed and/or printed immediately at the searcher's terminal. For larger numbers of retrieved abstracts, the search results usually are printed at a central computer location and mailed to the scientists the next day. Since early 1980, all abstracts have been indexed with a controlled vocabulary developed by the National Library of Medicine called Medical Subject Headings, or MeSH. This new indexing tool will be available for searching in 1982 and should facilitate the retrieval of information on specific requested topics.

The CANCERLIT database is used extensively. In 1980, searchers spent over 6,000 "connect hours" searching the CANCERLIT database. In addition to the tens of thousands of searches and citations printed or viewed at local terminals, records show that over 345,000 pages of printouts with about 802,000 citations were printed at the central computer location. The time and effort that would have been expended to locate the same information by manual search methods staggers the imagination.

One of the most convenient ways of using the data in CANCERLIT is through use of an automatic SDI (Selective Dissemination of Information) service that provides customized monthly updates on new literature from CANCERLIT. Investigators can obtain this service by discussing their special information needs with their biomedical librarian, who will develop a strategy for a monthly search of CANCERLINE. Every month, the investigator will receive automatically a printout listing the latest literature relevant to the requested areas of research. The search strategy can be modified by adding or deleting search terms so that the retrieved data more accurately meet the needs of the investigator. Since the abstracts included in the printouts of the SDI service are selected from the 4,000 new abstracts added to CANCERLIT each month, this service is equivalent to searching 3,000 biomedical journals monthly for newly published results in a specific area of research. The cost for this service is very small, and there is no charge for storing the search in the computer.

To our knowledge, the only other database that specifically focuses on cancer literature is CANCERNET, at the Institute Gustave-Roussy in Villejuif, France. This database is updated monthly, contains 15,000 records, and is growing at a rate of 12,000 records per year. The records contain complete bibliographic information but do not provide abstracts. CANCERNET is available for online searching through most European telecommunications systems. Input is provided by several cooperating countries, including Germany, Yugoslavia, and Italy. SDI services are also available to CANCERNET users.

ICRDB Publications

The most excellent and comprehensive collection of information is of little practical use unless it is readily available to those who can benefit from it. Databases are valuable sources of archival information. However, to be most useful, new information must be rapidly and actively disseminated directly to researchers in a convenient format on a continuing basis. This is achieved by several series of ICRDB publications containing information that is carefully selected, analyzed, and organized by experts. Input from subject specialists and active researchers ensures that each publication presents logically organized information that is more likely to meet the needs of the group of cancer researchers to which it is targeted.

The major ICRDB publications include: *The Compilation of Experimental Cancer Therapy Protocol Summaries,* derived from the CLINPROT database; the *Special Listings of Current Cancer Research Projects,* which are prepared from the CANCERLIT database; and *Cancergrams* and *Oncology Overviews,* which are prepared from the CANCERLIT database. The relationship of these publications to the ICRDB databases is shown in Figure 3-1.

The *Compilation of Experimental Cancer Therapy Protocol Summaries* contains a subset of the protocols in the CLINPROT database. Outlines of active Phase II and Phase III clinical protocols are listed under 15 different sections, each covering a major organ site or type of cancer. Protocols closed to patient entry during the preceding year are listed in abbreviated form, as are Phase I protocols activated during that period. The 1981 edition contained information on some 1,500 active protocols, 175 closed protocols, and 36 Phase I studies.

Complete and detailed tumor and agent indexes make it easy for clinicians to identify protocols for treating specific types of cancer and to identify tumor types being treated with a specific anticancer agent or combination of agents. In addition, the name, address, and telephone number of the study group chairperson or principal investigator is included for each protocol summary, to facilitate direct personal communication among research clinicians.

The *Compilation* is used by clinicians who design new protocols, who need to identify protocols for patient referral, or who would like to keep abreast of the entire spectrum of experimental protocols currently under way throughout the world. An updated edition of the *Compilation* is prepared in the first quarter of each new year and may be requested from the ICRDB Program. Complimentary copies of the *Compilation* are provided to some 6,000 research clinicians world-wide who request a copy after being notified that an updated issue is available.

The ICRDB Program also publishes a series of volumes known as *Special Listings of Current Cancer Research Projects*, which describe research currently under way around the world. Each of the 55 issues published annually covers a major cancer research topic, as illustrated by the representative sample of available *Special Listings* titles in Table 3-2. Collectively, they cover all aspects of the cancer research effort. Within each *Special Listing*, 100 to 500 project descriptions are organized into logical subcategories so that busy researchers easily can locate and review projects most closely related to their area of research. Most descriptions outline the objectives, experimental approach, and recent progress to date.

To disseminate most efficiently the collected information on worldwide cancer research activities, the ICRDB Program automatically sends *Special Listings* to both principal investigators and co-investigators working in the specific field covered by a given *Special Listing*. The wide availability of this information about ongoing research projects in 85 countries around the world is expected to promote timely collaboration among investigators and to avoid unnecessary duplication of research studies.

Cancergrams, another unique publication series of ICRDB, help cancer researchers keep abreast of the published literature. So voluminous and diffuse is the cancer literature of today, that individual researchers no longer can expect to keep abreast by relying upon yesterday's manual methods of information retrieval. *Cancergrams* utilize present-day information technology to distill, and rapidly deliver directly to the investigator's desk, the recently published results of cancer research.

Cancergrams in 66 different topic areas collectively cover the entire spectrum of cancer research. Representative *Cancergram* titles are given in Table 3-3. The raw material for each *Cancergram* is a batch of computer-selected abstracts of published articles, books, and so forth, received in the library during the previous month. These are screened rapidly to select the most significant and relevant abstracts for each *Cancergram* topic and then are sorted into logical

Table 3-2

Representative Titles of *Special Listings of Current Cancer Research Projects*

Cancer Sites: Etiology, Epidemiology, Diagnosis, Treatment Series
    Breast Cancer: Diagnosis, Prognosis, and Treatment
    Gynecologic Cancer: Etiology, Epidemiology, Diagnosis, and Therapy
    Male Reproductive System Neoplasms
    Endocrine Neoplasms: Epidemiology, Etiology, and Related Biology
    Oral and Head and Neck Cancer
    Etiology, Epidemiology, and Related Biology of Cancer of the Lower Respiratory Tract
    Bone and Cartilage Tumors and Soft-Tissue Sarcomas
    Clinical, Preclinical, and Basic Studies of Nervous System and Related Tumors
    Etiology, Epidemiology, and Biology of Melanomas and Other Skin Cancers

Clinical Diagnosis and Treatment Methods, and Preclinical Studies Series
    Clinical Diagnostic Radiology and Radiation Therapy
    Clinical and Experimental Cancer Immunotherapy
    Cancer Patient Supportive Care and Management
    Interferon and Other Anticancer and Antiviral Drugs

Carcinogenesis: Etiologic Factors and Mechanisms Series
    Nitroso Compounds
    The Relationship of Viruses to Human Cancer
    Genetics and Molecular Biology of DNA Tumor Viruses
    Effects of Chemical Carcinogens on Nucleic Acids, Proteins, and Chromosomes
    Modification of Chemical Carcinogenesis in Model Systems
    Occupational and Environmental Carcinogenesis

Cancer Biology/Immunology Series
    Tumor Immunogenetics and Related Transplantation Biology
    Tumor Immunology: Function and Characterization of Immune Cells and Antibodies
    Cell Differentiation, Tumor Growth, Invasion, and Metastasis
    Differentiation and Maturation of Normal and Neoplastic Hematopoietic Cells
    Development and Application of In Vitro Techniques

---

subject categories by scientists at three Cancer Information Dissemination and Analysis Centers (CIDACs). Each *Cancergram* series is prepared under the supervision of a consultant reviewer who is presently an active researcher in the subject area of that *Cancergram.* Review of every issue by these consultants ensures that *Cancergrams* will continue to reflect accurately the current status and emerging trends in each research area.

More than 10,500 scientists (chiefly principal investigators of cancer research projects) in 80 countries regularly receive *Cancergrams,* and they often circulate their *Cancergrams* among colleagues. Thus, the *Cancergram* service can have a profound and global impact on the progress of cancer research, since it provides the equivalent of a tailored literature search of a 3,000-journal "library" to several thousand researchers worldwide.

The fourth major ICRDB publication, *Oncology Overviews,* contains

Table 3-3

Representative Titles of *Cancergrams*

Cancer Diagnosis and Therapy Series (21 titles)
    Cancer Detection and Management Subseries
        Biological Markers
        Diagnostic Radiology
        Nuclear Medicine
    Diagnosis, Treatment Subseries (13 titles, focusing on various cancer sites)
    Clinical Cancer Immunology and Immunotherapy
    Pediatric Oncology
    Rehabilitation and Supportive Care
    Clinical Treatment of Cancer—Radiation Therapy

Chemical, Environmental and Radiation Carcinogenesis Series (21 titles)
    Dietary Aspects of Carcinogenesis
    Environmental and Occupational Carbinogenesis
    Hormonal Carcinogenesis
    Radiation Carcinogenesis
    Organ Site Carcinogenesis Subseries (7 titles, focusing on various cancer sites)
    Modification of Carcinogenesis
    Mechanisms of Carcinogenesis Subseries
        Activation and Metabolism of Carcinogens
        Macromolecular Alteration and Repair
        Oncogenic Transformation

Cancer Virology/Immunology/Biology Series (24 titles)
    Antitumor and Antiviral Agents Subseries
        Mechanism of Action
        Experimental Therapeutics, Toxicology, and Pharmacology
    Oncofetal Proteins
    Virus Studies in Humans and Other Primates
    Viral Immunology
    Hormones in Cancer-Related Biology Subseries
        Steroid Hormones
        Nonsteroid Hormones
    Immunobiology and Cancer Subseries
        Tumor-Associated Antigens
        Functional Aspects of Cellular Immunity

---

retrospective reviews of research on cancer topics, specially selected for high current interest. Each issue provides 100 to 500 abstracts of the most significant research results published during the last few years and includes an editorial commentary contributed by a consultant reviewer who is a recognized expert in the field. Abstracts are selected and organized by the staffs of the CIDACs, mentioned previously, who develop the *Overviews* in close collaboration with the consultant reviewers. These publications provide a convenient mechanism by which cancer researchers can rapidly acquire necessary background and become conversant with emerging research areas of high interest.

A representative sample of available *Oncology Overview* titles is listed in Table 3-4. These *Oncology Overviews* are disseminated to primary authors who recently have published articles in the subject area of the publication, and to principal investigators who are conducting research in the field. Complimentary copies of these retrospective bibliographies also are made available to researchers upon request. Young investigators who are entering an area of research recently covered by an *Oncology Overview* will find this publication indispensable both for identifying key scientists working in the field and for quickly reviewing major substantive articles in the subject area.

Special International Projects

To accelerate the rapid transfer of new cancer research technology between countries, a special project called the International Cancer Research Technology Transfer Program (ICRETT) was developed. The ICRETT Program supports cancer researchers who collaborate for a brief period of time with a scientist in a different country to learn, develop, or verify new techniques. This project

Table 3-4
Representative Titles of *Oncology Overviews*

Cancer Diagnosis and Therapy Series
    Nutritional Therapy for the Cancer Patient
    Radionuclide Bone Scans in the Diagnosis and Staging of Cancer
    Nitroheterocyclic Compounds as Hypoxic Cell Radiosensitizers
    Intra-arterial Chemotherapy
    Malignant Pleural Effusions
    Supportive Care of the Cancer Patient: Management of Infections and
        Hematologic Complications

Carcinogenesis Series
    Chemoprevention of Carcinogenesis
    Genetic Predisposition to Cancer in Man
    Age-Related Factors Which May Predispose to Carcinogenesis
    The Role of Dietary Nitrate and Nitrite in Human Carcinogenesis
    Short-Term Tests for Potential Mutagens and Carcinogens Subseries (6 titles)
    Dioxins and Dibenzofurans in Carcinogenesis

Cancer Virology/Immunology/Biology Series
    Virus Latency and Oncogenesis
    Hepatitis B Virus
    Interferon Subseries (3 titles)
    Role of Proteases in Metastasis
    Ectopic Hormones and Enzymes
    Cell Hybridization
    Viral Transforming Proteins

is administered by the International Union Against Cancer (UICC), with the help of a panel of international experts who review applications and recommend selection of individuals to receive support. To date, some 500 investigators from 43 countries have benefited from the support of such collaborative projects.

While improved awareness and communication among individual cancer researchers is the ultimate goal of all ICRDB activities, some of the best strategies toward achieving this goal have included international collaboration among cancer research organizations. Worldwide exchange of epidemiology data is promoted by the International Clearinghouse for Ongoing Research in Cancer Epidemiology, which is operated by two international cancer organizations. Under this collaborative project, the International Agency for Research on Cancer in Lyon, France, contacts epidemiologists in all parts of the world requesting descriptions of current epidemiological research projects. These descriptions are entered into a database at the German Cancer Research Center in Heidelberg, published in an annual *Directory of Ongoing Research in Cancer Epidemiology,*[2] and entered into the CANCERPROJ database. This *Directory* and epidemiology clearinghouse operation are particularly important, since they provide a means by which scientists can identify other investigators working in similar areas of epidemiology research and share ideas, arrange for collaboration, and avoid duplication of studies that have been or are being carried out by others.

Early in the development of the ICRDB Program, the Latin American Cancer Research Information Program (LACRIP) was established to promote the collection and dissemination of information in Latin America. LACRIP is operated by the Pan American Health Organization in cooperation with its regional library of medicine in São Paulo. Major LACRIP activities include the screening and selection of cancer-related articles published in Latin America and the collection of descriptions of current research projects, including cancer therapy protocols, from Latin American researchers. Through a special information program, cancer information is disseminated automatically to more than 3,600 scientists within Latin America by means of 15 current awareness bulletins issued four times a year. They contain abstracts describing recent progress in clinical areas of interest to Latin American scientists. In addition, requests for information and literature searches from Latin American scientists are channeled through the LACRIP staff, who provide computer-generated printouts of abstracts that address the individual requests.

One of the most important accomplishments of the LACRIP was the establishment of a Collaborative Cancer Treatment Research Program (CCTRP), which involves close collaboration among clinical oncologists at eight cancer centers in the United States and nine centers in Latin America. This project provides a very effective mechanism for rapid dissemination of current cancer treatment methodology throughout Latin America and serves as an excellent model that could be extended to other countries.

The ICRDB Program supports a Committee for International Collaborative Activities (CICA) within the framework of the International Union Against Cancer (UICC). The membership of CICA consists of the directors of major cancer research centers from 15 different countries. Major CICA activities include making arrangements and providing liaison needed to support the international collection of cancer research project descriptions and collecting data for an *International Directory of Specialized Cancer Research and Treatment Establishments,*[3] which is revised and updated every few years.

UICC/CICA also was directly responsible for catalyzing the formation of an Organization of European Cancer Institutes (OECI) and an Organization of Latin American Cancer Institutes. These new organizations, along with other UICC/CICA-initiated activities, provide the basis for increased collaboration and liaison among cancer researchers in many countries throughout the world.

A serious impediment to the worldwide exchange and application of clinical cancer research findings has been the absence of standardized data-reporting procedures. This has made it extremely difficult for clinicians to compare effectively the results of studies conducted at different institutions within a country or at institutions in various countries. Thus, an especially significant achievement of the UICC/CICA was the development of an International Cancer Patient Data Exchange System (ICPDES), which made available to clinical oncologists, for the first time, a mechanism for the collection of standardized, uniform data on cancer patients from many countries. As of May 1981, data have been entered into ICPDES on 20,070 cancer patients from nine countries, including Russia.

The ICPDES was modeled after a similar system called the Centralized Cancer Patient Data System (CCPDS), which initially was developed and supported by the ICRDB Program and the American Association of Cancer Institutes for collection of cancer patient data in the United States. The CCPDS currently contains uniform data on more than 100,000 patients from 21 cancer centers. A major and lasting benefit of these clinical data projects is the increased effort and attention devoted to the collection and analysis of uniform clinical data at many of the cancer centers throughout the world and the resulting improvement of procedures for processing clinical data.

The ICRDB Program has provided support for several World Health Organization projects that have brought us closer to achieving the goal of worldwide uniform reporting of clinical data. Among these is a project that resulted in the development and publication of an international coded nomenclature for neoplasms, entitled *The International Classification of Diseases for Oncology (ICD-0).*[4] This detailed coding system for the histopathology and anatomical sites of neoplasms was designed for use in tumor registries, cancer data banks, pathology laboratories, and departments of vital statistics. The *ICD-0* has been published in English, Spanish, Portuguese, Russian, French, and German and is widely used for patient data-collection systems.

Another project carried out by the World Health Organization and supported in part by the ICRDB Program has resulted in a series of some 25 publications entitled the *International Histological Classification of Tumors.* These books, distributed by the World Health Organization, also are designed to promote the worldwide adoption of uniform and standardized criteria for the diagnosis and classification of neoplasms

An *International Histological Classification of Tumors of Domestic Animals,* developed by the Armed Forces Institute of Pathology in collaboration with the World Health Organization, also was supported by the ICRDB Program. This project included the preparation, duplication, and distribution of veterinary pathology slides and related materials to veterinary schools and other cancer research groups worldwide.

Summary

In response to a congressional mandate, the ICRDB Program has developed a comprehensive model system to collect cancer information and to disseminate it to researchers throughout the world. This multifaceted, international approach includes the establishment and maintenance of specialized cancer databases, the production of several series of technical publications, and the support of activities by international organizations that stimulate the worldwide exchange of information and promote the standardized reporting of clinical data. Every effort has been made to collect information that accurately represents the research activity carried out worldwide. Advanced science information technology has been used to provide the collected information to researchers on a timely basis.

The availability of this comprehensive range of technical cancer information services to scientists in multiple, readily accessible, and convenient formats is felt to have a significant impact on the efficiency and productivity of cancer research and is believed to promote increased communication and collaboration among basic and clinical investigators throughout the world.

References

1. U.S. Department of Health and Human Services, Public Health Service, *Directory of Cancer Research Information Resources.* Washington, DC, National Institutes of Health, National Cancer Institute, 1981.
2. Muir CS, Wagner G (eds), *Directory of On-Going Research in Cancer Epidemiology.* Lyon, France, International Agency for Research on Cancer, World Health Organization, 1981.

3. Committee for International Collaborative Activities, *International Directory of Specialized Cancer Research and Treatment Establishments,* ed. 2. Geneva, Switzerland. International Union Against Cancer, 1978, vol 33.

4. World Health Organization, *The International Classification of Diseases for Oncology (ICD-O).* Geneva, Switzerland, World Health Organization, 1976.

II

Cancer Treatment
and Humanism

4

The Development and Practice of Oncology

Ronald W. Raven

Oncology is a multidisciplinary subject composed of the different arts and sciences concerned with the cause, prevention, diagnosis, and treatment of the large group of diseases known as cancer throughout many centuries. Since the majority of these diseases are serious and often fatal, the name "cancer" causes considerable fear and pessimism in the minds of many people. "Cancer" is not a precise scientific term, because it designates many diseases with different causation and manifestations that require various treatment modalities. Their prognosis also is very uneven. These are good reasons to discard the term "cancer" and to substitute the term "oncological diseases."

The emergence of oncology is a major advance in medicine, for it provides us with a vehicle to correlate knowledge concerning all these diseases from basic oncological sciences and to synthesize new knowledge from laboratory and clinical research. This multidisciplinary subject thus brings together researchers, clinicians, and members of other caring professions to establish teamwork with the ultimate objective of preventing these diseases and mitigating the suffering and saving the lives of afflicted patients (Raven, 1975).

Evolution of Knowledge

In far-off millenia, cancer was rare and many nonmalignant swellings in the body were thus classified. They included innocent tumors, in addition to swellings caused by injuries and inflammation. Information is very scanty about these conditions, and we rely on the Egyptian papyruses for descriptions of tumors found in mummies. There are few descriptions of malignant tumors until the time of Hippocrates (460 to 370 B.C.). Hippocrates and his school contributed to our knowledge by attempting to develop a classification of tumors based upon facts derived from observation (Hippocrates, 1839-1861). We still are searching for improved systems of classification of tumors and the stages of malignant disease.

Progress after Hippocrates was slow: About three centuries elapsed before the next advances were made by Aulus Cornelius Celsus (25 B.C. to A.D. 50), who lived in Rome, the great center of Western civilization at that time. He distinguished benign from malignant tumors and described their progression in stages (Celsus, 1935-1938). The advent of Clarissimus (or Claudius) Galen (A.D. 130 to 200), born in Pergamon in Asia Minor, ushered in a new and prolonged epoch, for he exercised a profound influence on medicine for a millenium. He, like Hippocrates, enunciated the humoral theory of cancer (Galen, 1824), for he considered that tumors were caused by an excess of black bile, which tended to solidify in certain parts of the body, as the lip, tongue, and breast, where tumors then developed. This theory was superseded later, when others including E. I. K. Virchow (1847) propounded the theory of local irritation and Julius Cohnheim (1877-1880) advanced the theory of embryonal rests.

It is noteworthy how greatly progress was impeded for centuries by the lack of scientific instruments and methodology. Increasing knowledge was dependent upon clinical observation of patients with accurate descriptions of tumors. The development of the microscope by Johannes Müller (1838) enabled him to classify tumors according to their cellular structure, and this stimulated further speculative thought about their causation.

For many centuries knowledge about cancer was meager and the subject was shrouded in mysticism and ignorance. There were, however, periods of illumination when the light streamed in and decisive advances were made. In 1775, Percivall Pott, the London surgeon, published his important observation that skin cancer is common in chimney sweeps, where the disease develops from skin contamination by soot. Another advance came when Yamagiwa and Itchikawa (1917) in Japan produced epithelioma in the skin of the rabbit's ear by applying coal tar. This vital sequence was brought to its brilliant conclusion when Sir Ernest Kennaway and his colleagues (Kennaway, Cook, Hieger, & Mayneord, 1932) published their work at the Cancer Hospital, now The Royal Marsden Hospital and Institute of Cancer Research, London, announcing the isolation and synthesis of the pentacyclic hydrocarbon 3-4-benzpyrene and correlating its chemical structure with carcinogenicity. This is the first synthetic chemical known to produce cancer—a chemical carcinogen. We now recognize a long range of chemicals, both inorganic and organic, that possess this property. They include arsenic, nitrosamines, asbestos, vinylchloride, and many others. Other carcinogens include various radiations, such as solar rays, x-rays, and rays produced by nuclear fission. While so many carcinogens now are recognized, we still do not know the exact mechanism that results in cancer.

The Broad Imagery of Oncology

The field of oncology comprises all knowledge concerning the nature, causation, and behavior of the oncological diseases. The practice of oncology includes the methods of prevention, diagnosis, and treatment of these diseases.

There is continual growth within the many divisions of oncology, with a constant feedback of new knowledge, especially from research oncology into clinical oncology, so that less delay occurs before patients benefit from new discoveries.

Research Oncology

Laboratory

This discipline developed in the twentieth century, when transplantable and induced tumors in animals became available for study. Reference was made to carcinogenesis as a key subject where natural and synthetic carcinogens are of tremendous practical importance in national prevention programs. Increasing attention now is given to transplacental and intrauterine carcinogenesis, with the object of preventing these diseases in children.

Attention was directed to the possibility that neoplasms are caused by viruses when Francis Peyton Rous (1910) described the chicken sarcoma (Rous sarcoma), which is transmissible by cell-free filtrates or dessicates. The virus theory was developed further by William Ewart Gye (1925), who postulated the combination of a virus with an intrinsic chemical factor to produce the Rous sarcoma.

While it is known that a virus can produce animal tumors, there is no proof yet to demonstrate that any human malignant tumor is of viral origin. Endocrinology is making important academic and practical contributions in association with steroid chemistry. The discovery of cytoplasmic substances called estrogen receptors, which bind and transfer estrogens into the cell nuclei where estrogen function is exercised, is an important advance, as it can predict the response of breast carcinoma to hormonal therapy. The clinical results, in advanced carcinoma of the breast and in carcinoma of the prostate, from manipulating the hormone control system can be very impressive. More research is required to understand the mechanism of these systems.

During recent decades, tremendous interest has developed in molecular biology and immunology of tumors, for we now recognize that defense mechanisms exist in the body that are able to destroy potentially malignant cells, mechanisms that are related to tumor-specific antigens. Immunology is concerned not only with tumor development but also with growth rates, metastasis, and the clinical state of patients. Methods are being sought to stimulate patients' defense mechanisms to overcome these diseases. This immunotherapy, however, has not yet been established; eventually it may be used most effectively in conjunction with surgery and other therapies. The biggest advance for these diseases would be immuno-prophylaxis similar to all the great killer diseases that have been prevented by vaccination, inoculation, and other therapies.

Here we have a glimpse of the broad spectrum of laboratory research that is proceeding all over the world in an attempt to wrest from nature these difficult secrets of neoplasia.

Clinical

For many centuries our knowledge about cancer was based entirely on clinical observations. In addition to the chimney sweeps' skin cancer described by Percivall Pott, another important observation was made by the German urologist, Rehn (1895), concerning patients with bladder carcinoma who had worked in the manufacture of the dye magenta from commercial aniline. Following this publication were many reports of industrial bladder tumors occurring in countries with a chemical dye industry. This stimulated laboratory and field research to determine which chemical or chemicals are most dangerous. Case (1966) carried out the most detailed work in this area, examining large numbers of hospital records and reports, concluding that the chemical 2-naphthylamine is the most dangerous chemical of the research sample used.

Epidemiology

There is considerable interest in knowing the geographical incidence of the oncological diseases in different nations throughout the world. No nation is immune, but there are considerable variations in different hemispheres and countries. For example, stomach carcinoma is common in Japan, whereas its incidence is falling in the United Kingdom and the United States. Breast carcinoma is very common in women of the Western world but is relatively infrequent in Japanese women. Carcinoma of the esophagus varies considerably, having a high incidence in the Transkei population of South Africa, in Iran, and in China. Primary malignant liver tumors are frequent in certain parts of Africa, especially in the Bantu population. The study of the geographical distribution of these diseases leads to the identification of etiological factors. The identification of the "tobacco cancers," chiefly of the lung but also occurring in the mouth, larynx, pharynx, and urinary bladder, is an outstanding achievement. The reduction or abolition of tobacco usage is probably the biggest single challenge for preventive medicine, as the incidence of lung cancer is now so high as to constitute an epidemic. More research is required for a better understanding of the role of alcohol in cancer, especially carcinoma of the esophagus. Our lifestyle, habits, and customs must be examined in detail so that the appropriate adjustments can be made to avoid cancer.

Research and clinical oncologists must work together to provide for the transmission of ideas and knowledge. The past delays in applying new discoveries for the prevention and treatment of other diseases should not be repeated with the oncological diseases.

Clinical Oncology

The prevention, diagnosis, and treatment of patients with the oncological diseases is a task of considerable magnitude and responsibility. A specialist no longer can work in isolation; a complete team is essential. This team includes medical, surgical, and radiation oncologists; pathologists; hospital and community physicians and family doctors; medical social workers; psychologists; physiotherapists; occupational and speech therapists; and chaplains. Regular joint consultation clinics are necessary when definitive treatment is arranged and an efficient system of continuing care and follow-up is defined.

The assessment and management of these patients has made enormous progress during recent years, so that considerable specialist knowledge and involvement are required. Clinical expertise is required in the use of sophisticated techniques, including endoscopy; radiology, including tomography and xerography; scintiscans; computerized axial tomography; and ultrasonography. Laboratory investigations involve the subfields of hematology, biochemistry, immunology, and histopathology. The clinical oncologist works closely with colleagues in these diagnostic and pathology disciplines and with other clinical specialists.

Clinical oncologists all require a sound basic knowledge of the theory of oncology, which is acquired by a continuing learning process throughout professional life. Oncological sciences are growing continually so that constant study of the relevant related literature and attendance at seminars and special courses are necessary to keep up to date.

Training of the Clinical Oncologist

The education of the clinical oncologist is a continuous learning process that requires broad knowledge encompassing the numerous scientific disciplines. The real objective of training is to develop fine clinical judgment and technical skills for the investigation, diagnosis, treatment, and continuing care of patients with oncological diseases. The skills of surgical, medical, and radiation treatment are different, yet complementary. Surgical, medical, and radiation oncologists must recognize the indications for each treatment modality, either alone or combined. The medical oncologist first must be a competent, trained, and well-rounded physician before specializing in oncology. The radiation oncologist must undergo a sound training in general medicine before undergoing a longer period of specialist training in radiation techniques. Surgery is currently the major treatment modality for these diseases and is likely to remain so in the foreseeable future. The development of oncological operations during a period of less than a century forms a major and brilliant part of the whole history of surgery. These masters of surgery who designed these classical operations, shown in Table 4-1, carried out their work without the tremendous help we have today with regard to skilled nursing, anesthesia, antibacterial chemicals, rehabilitation techniques, and the facilities provided in postoperative and intensive care units.

At the present time, and until there is a sufficient number of surgical oncologists trained to carry out this heavy workload, general and specialist surgeons will continue to be responsible for the management of large numbers of patients with oncological diseases, in addition to dealing with other general surgical conditions. Many surgeons have a special interest in surgical oncology and serve a very valuable role. It is likely that the specialized medical treatment of these diseases will expand in the future, with more academic departments being developed, especially in surgical and medical oncology.

Academic departments have an important bridging function between oncology and other clinical academic departments, in addition to their clinical work, teaching, training, and research programs. They function as important catalysts of oncological knowledge. Systematic teaching of all aspects of oncology is developing, both for graduates and undergraduates. Suitable courses of integrative oncological instruction should be organized in all our medical schools.

Table 4-1
Major Oncological Operations

Surgeon	Year	Operation
Billroth	1881	Subtotal Gastrectomy
Halsted	1890	Radical Mastectomy
Schlatter	1897	Total Gastrectomy
Von Mickulicz	1898	Esophagogastrectomy
Werthheim	1900	Radical Hysterectomy
Miles	1908	Abdominoperineal Excision of Rectum
Torek	1913	Esophagectomy
Trotter	1913	Partial Pharyngectomy
Graham & Singer	1933	Pneumonectomy

Basic Sciences in Oncology

Pathology

Pathology now consists of many laboratory sciences, including clinical chemistry, hematology, histopathology, cytology, medical microbiology, immunology, and virology. Studies of particular value focus on the general pathology and functional properties of tumors and their modes of spread into contiguous tissues and through the lymphatics and blood stream. The presence of tumors in the body causes a disturbance in the metabolic and immunological systems, which must be understood clearly in the management of patients.

Hematology

In the clinical care of cancer patients, hematological investigations can be lifesaving. Support therapy, especially cell component therapy, is usually required; so that principles of blood storage, the indications for various transfusions, and the treatment techniques must be learned. Allogenic bone marrow grafting is used increasingly and requires a knowledge of histocompatibility. Patients, especially those undergoing chemotherapy, develop an immune suppression where microbiological infections flourish. This may be lethal and requires careful management.

Biochemistry

The biochemical changes in these patients are numerous and complicated, for which an increasing number of investigations is available to provide a complete biochemical profile. The recognition of special syndromes and the instant correction of the biochemical abnormalities also can be life-saving. A good example is the hypercalcemia that may develop with carcinoma metastases in the skeleton. Biochemical abnormalities occur frequently in patients who are undergoing medical therapy or a major surgical operation, so these patients require constant biochemical monitoring. Detection of abnormalities such as alphafetoprotein and carcinoembryonic antigen may lead to the diagnosis of tumors such as liver and colonic carcinoma. These tests give encouragement for the further development of immunodiagnosis in the future.

The subject of carcinogenesis, including chemical carcinogenesis, is of profound importance. The mechanism of carcinogenesis, including the activation and binding of carcinogens, is under constant investigation.

Endocrinology and Metabolic Medicine

A strong relationship exists between the endocrine system and neoplasia. A number of tumors secrete ectopic hormones, which cause clinical syndromes. These syndromes can be recognized, thereby leading to the diagnosis of the secretory tumor. Good examples are tumors of the lung and the adrenal, and pituitary glands. Our knowledge of these ectopic hormones is increasing constantly. Tumors such as carcinoma of the breast and prostate are hormone dependent. Remarkable regression results in about 50 percent of patients with breast carcinoma by manipulation of the hormonal control systems, by the administration of synthetic hormones, or by removal of the ovaries and adrenal glands. Men with prostatic carcinoma can remain symptom-free for many years by the administration of synthetic estrogen. Considerable research concerning these hormonal control systems has been generated. Already, hormone receptors have been identified in tumors which indicate whether the patient is likely to benefit from hormonal treatment.

Immunology and Tumor Biology

Many patients remain free of recurrent and metastatic disease from a primary malignant tumor for many years and then, quite suddenly, extensions of the disease may manifest themselves. This appears to be due to a final breakdown in the resistance of patients due to some immunological failure. It is also well known that malignant tumors can regress, either partially or completely, without active treatment. This biological phenomenon is of obvious importance, for it is most likely associated with an immunological mechanism. Methods to stimulate the immune process designed to enable patients to overcome their tumors are now being sought, but we cannot yet speak of tumor immunotherapy. Immunological techniques are developing in tumor diagnosis, such as the identification of the carcinoembryonic antigen (CEA) in colon carcinoma and in neuroblastoma in children, and alphafetoprotein (AFP) in hepatocellular carcinoma. It is possible that, in the future, immunoprophylaxis will be available by the administration of vaccines or sera and malignant disease may be prevented as have been other lethal diseases, such as typhoid fever, diphtheria, and smallpox.

Genetics

Genetic mechanisms occupy an important place in our understanding of oncological diseases, and the knowledge about them is expanding rapidly. Immunogenetics and cytogenetics are established disciplines that contribute to the care of patients. We now recognize that certain rare neoplasms are of genetic inheritance, and, where there is a familial disease, members of these families who desire offspring may seek guidance from genetic counselors.

Clinical Pharmacology

There is now a wide range of chemicals that are beneficial, or even curative, when used in treating oncological diseases. They usually are given in combination, according to carefully designed protocols. Chemotherapy often is combined with surgery and radiotherapy. It is essential to understand the pharmacology of these chemicals, for they have important side-effects from which patients must be protected. This subject is of special importance to the medical oncologist, but all physicians who use these potent chemicals must be familiar with their dosage schedules, metabolism, and excretion, in addition to understanding their indications, limitations, toxicity, and chemical interactions.

Radiobiology

Radiobiological research has contributed much to the radiotherapy of oncological diseases and is of special importance to the radiation oncologist, who should work in close collaboration with the radiobiologist. To a lesser extent, this also is necessary for the medical oncologist. A good understanding of cell kinetics is needed, including the characterization of normal and neoplastic cells, the cell cycle and cellular division, cell loss and multiplication, and the mechanism of cellular repair.

Radiation Physics

All clinical oncologists, but especially radiation oncologists, need to understand the principles of radiation physics. This includes the physics of ionizing radiation and its interaction with cells, tissues, and materials. This is the basis of safe, accurate, and effective radiotherapy for oncological diseases.

Epidemiology

This subject is of profound interest to all oncologists, and an essential part of their continuing education throughout professional life. There is tremendous interest in the world geographical distribution and incidence of neoplastic disease. Important studies show different sex, age, racial, and occupational incidence, in addition to different rates of development of neoplasia in migrant populations. The relationship between carcinogenesis and various social and ethnic habits and customs is also being studied actively. The clinical oncologist must be familiar with epidemiological methodology, including taking population surveys, framing questionnaires, compiling clinical case records, and using tumor registries.

Medical Statistics

This subject includes the design of clinical trials, data recording and sampling, and the scientific use of controls. It is necessary to be familiar with the different techniques for presenting data, measuring mortality, and the use of life tables. The clinical oncologist must always seek better methods of treatment based on the latest survival rates and other assessments of present therapy.

Related Subspecialties within Oncology

Gerontology

This science is concerned with the process of aging and its effect on organs and tissues, and it embraces the pathology of senescence. There is a known age relationship of various neoplasms; for example, mesodermal tumors are more common in childhood, while carcinomas usually are found in older adults. Carcinogenesis is proportional to the exposure time, for there may be a long latent period, as much as 25 years and more, between the first application of a carcinogen and the clinical manifestation of a malignant tumor. Carcinogenic effects are manifested as successive mutations.

Anthropology

This science must be included, for it is the science of humanity in its widest sense, where humans are studied in their environment. These studies embrace humanity in different cultures with various beliefs about health, illness, and treatment modalities. Account is taken also of group behavior and group communications, which are important features in understanding the doctor–patient relationship.

Pediatric Oncology

Special centers for this established science are available in which children with these diseases are investigated and treated. This is an important development because there are difficult and idiosyncratic clinical pediatric problems to solve.

Gynecological Oncology

This science deals with neoplastic diseases in the female pelvis. Collaboration with radiation oncology is needed for combined treatment.

Head and Neck Oncology

Many neoplastic diseases in the head and neck present particularly complex and special problems to solve. This requires teamwork among surgical, medical, and radiation oncologists, in addition to collaboration with plastic surgeons, dentists, and other specialists for diagnosis and general management. Advances have been made in special centers where head and neck surgical oncologists work closely with colleagues, with access to all the requisite facilities.

Nursing Oncology

This is a relatively new and quickly developing discipline that already has received international recognition. Nurses have an important role in clinical oncology, both in the hospital and in the community. Hospital nurses must keep abreast of new and sophisticated methods of treatment, which requires specialized education and training in oncology. Many patients are treated in intensive care units and need constant nurse observation and monitoring. Nurses must be familiar with the principles and objectives of different treatment modalities, in addition to their side-effects. It must be noted that nursing observation and care is often a round-the-clock task. In certain cases, nurses rarely leave their patients. In this exacting work, great patience, sympathy, and understanding are essential to deal not only with the patients' physical condition, but also with their personal and spiritual needs. In particular, nursing of dying patients requires sensitive understanding and skillful support.

In the community, the role of nurses is important for the continuing care of patients in collaboration with family doctors. The Marie Curie Memorial Foundation has an organized Day and Night Domiciliary Nursing Service that is nationwide in the United Kingdom. The nurses take care of patients in their homes and stay with them day and night, according to their needs. This service has proved to be of tremendous value throughout many years, for both patients and their families.

Nurses also play an important role in educating the public about preventing the oncological diseases and maintaining good health. They carry out valuable work in special detection centers where "well" people come for screening tests.

General Practice Oncology

Family doctors have an important role on oncology teams. A full description of this extensive work is not attempted here, but attention is drawn to various aspects. In the early diagnosis of oncological diseases, family doctors usually are the first medical professionals to contact patients. Initially the symptoms

often are indefinite and difficult for patients to describe; consequently, doctors must be on the alert for a serious disease. Following a careful clinical examination, a decision is made about investigations and referral to specialists. Family
doctors also are important in community health care systems, giving advice on
self-care and family-care, principles that are stressed in the wider field of public
education. Importance is placed on the prevention of oncological diseases, as
this is currently our greatest hope in the control of neoplastic diseases.

The needs of seriously ill patients nursed at home are considerable, and
family doctors take a vital part in their care. They have many distressing symptoms to ameliorate, of which pain of various grades is of outstanding importance. At this time the patient's family needs constant supportive help, and the
family doctor may collaborate with the clergy in giving this vital help. The importance of continuing care for the family during the testing time of bereavement is stressed, for the suffering caused by the loss of a loved one is considerable and calls for the most sensitive and sympathetic treatment by members of
the caring professions.

Social Oncology

This division of oncology embraces some of the most important and extensive
aspects of oncological work, which can be indicated only in brief outline here,
but this by no means diminishes its impact. In spite of its enormous applicability
today, the whole subject has tremendous future potential.

Prevention of the Oncological Diseases. This is our great future expectation for cancer control. Already 70 percent of these diseases are potentially
preventable. Prevention has a scientific basis that enables us to speak with as-
surance. It is not an emotional or hypothetical exercise, but a key solution to
this major health problem. Research has provided data about a wide range of
exogenous carcinogens of physical, chemical, and perhaps viral natures. We now
must learn how to protect ourselves from contamination by these agents and
how to avoid other circumstances that effect carcinogenesis. For instance, it
is important to reduce stress and strain, as it has been shown experimentally
that animals placed under stress are more liable to develop malignant tumors.
There are well-known hazards from radiation of various kinds, occupational
risks, and risks from habits and customs. The outstanding example is the great
risk from smoking tobacco. Increasing attention is rightly being given to the
protection of nonsmokers from exposure to tobacco smoke. There is, of course,
keen governmental awareness of this and other forms of carcinogenic contamination that can be prevented by the protection of food from pesticides and
chemical additives. An enlightened national program of prevention is essential
and must be supported by a strong, effective national effort. Both citizens
and government have responsible parts to play in order to secure the maximum
benefits.

Community Education and Counseling. It is necessary to carry out health education for the public. There are many ways of doing this work today through the various media, at meetings of specific groups of people, by family and individual counseling, and by other methods of education. Health education should begin with the young people in our schools. They would benefit from instruction in self-care, which forms part of their general knowledge of human biology. Voluntary organizations can make a most valuable contribution in this field by helping to inform the public about oncological diseases. This includes teaching preventive measures and providing information for the proper actions to be carried out, should the suspicious symptoms of cancer occur.

Rehabilitation. Patients with oncological diseases may be disabled in many ways. The object of rehabilitation is the restoration of the whole patient, spiritually and physically, to a life of longevity and good quality. Considerable help and support can be given to all these patients, even those suffering with advanced diseases.

There are three categories of patients with differing rehabilitation needs. First, many patients are cured and are able to resume their usual lives and work. Second, there are patients with a residual disability caused either by the disease or by its treatment, but this group can be fully rehabilitated. Third, there exists the group of patients with uncontrolled disease, various chronic disabilities, and a short life expectancy. Many, however, can be helped to become more self-supporting, for a time, thus shortening the period of total disability when they are completely dependent upon others.

The individual rehabilitation program for each patient is planned by the team at the time of diagnosis and is made to embrace both the definitive treatment in the hospital and the continuing care in the community. Many different professional skills are necessary, including patient counseling and family education. There are various nutritional and hematological abnormalities that are rectified by specific treatment.

There are at least four divisions of patients to be dealt with in the rehabilitation unit. First are the patients with major and minor amputations affecting limbs, breasts, and genitalia. Second are patients who have undergone excisional surgery involving the face, maxilla, mandible, larynx, pharynx, urinary bladder, and rectum. This introduced the need for stomal care, tracheostomy, ileal conduit, and colostomy. Third are patients who have undergone endocrine ablation, as of the thyroid, adrenal, and pituitary glands and who require replacement therapy. Fourth are patients with a major paralysis, tetreplegia, paraplegia, hemiplegia, or a cauda equina paralysis. No attempt is made here to describe all the care and treatment required by such seriously disabled patients and their families.

An important part of research rehabilitation is the provision of better prostheses for patients after various amputations and other excisional operations. Collaborative research between biomedical engineering and prosthetics is proceeding with this objective. Limb prostheses have reached high standards of appearance and function, and powered limbs now are being developed. There is a real need to provide a functional hand with more functional finger movements. Excellent prostheses are available as replacements for the facial soft tissues and the jaws. Following laryngectomy and laryngopharyngectomy, every effort is made through speech therapy to restore a speaking voice. When this remains unsatisfactory, pharynegeal vibrators are very helpful. Patients with paralyzed sphincters of the urinary bladder and anorectum suffer greatly with incontinence; electronic implants to restore sphincteric function now are being developed.

Research also is concerned with the body metabolism and the nutritional status of patients in whom these functions can be profoundly disturbed by oncological diseases. These abnormalities also are linked with cell-mediated immunity. The problem of pain is being studied extensively from different aspects, including its causation, biochemistry, and treatment. The discovery of brain opiates, the endorphins and encephalins, could lead eventually to their natural exploitation in pain relief, perhaps curtailing the need for injecting synthetic opiates. The role of vitamins in these diseases is imperfectly understood, although we are learning more about their importance. The ability of patients to undergo chemotherapy and radiotherapy is very dependent on their nutritional state, which must be brought up to, and maintained at, its optimum.

In the development of oncology, the subject of rehabilitation is of profound importance for patients following definitive treatment. Much effort and expertise are required to restore these patients to lives of good quality.

Resettlement. The final objective of the treatment of patients with oncological diseases is to resettle them in family life and enable them to return to work and independent living. Before patients return home it frequently is advisable to discuss their condition and needs with key members of the family, for certain readjustments may be required in human relationships and also in the physical conditions of the home. Actual visits to the family in the home can be very rewarding in finding solutions to various problems.

Resettlement of the patient at work is another matter. The patient may be able to resume usual activities and responsibilities. It has been shown that many patients treated successfully for oncological diseases can carry the same workload as the normal population, and their off-work hours are no higher. It may be necessary, however, for some adjustments to be made in the patient's work or for alternative employment to be found. Satisfactory solutions to all these resettlement problems enhance the quality of life for both the patient and the family.

Conclusion

The advent and development of oncology means the coming of a new dawn to dispel the darkness that has enshrouded this large group of serious diseases known for centuries as "cancer." It is with confidence that we can anticipate scientific and clinical developments in our knowledge and practice that most certainly will result in important advances in prevention, treatment, and cure.

References

Case, R. A. M. *Annals of the Royal College of Surgeons of England, 39,* 213, 1966.

Celsus, Aulus. *De Medicina.* 3 vols. W. G. Spencer (English trans.). London: Heinemann, 1935–1938.

Cohnheim, Julius F. *Vorlesungen über Allgemeine Pathologie.* 2 vols. Berlin: Hirschwald, 1877–1880.

Galen, Clarissimus. *De Tumoribus Praeter Naturam. Opera Omnia.* C. G. Kuhn (Ed.). Leipzig, 1824. 7:705–32.

Gye, W. E. Etiology of malignant new growths. *Lancet, 2,* 109, 1925.

Hippocrates. *Oeuvres completes d'Hippocrate. Traduction nouvelle avec le texte gree en regard.* 10 vols. E. Littre (trans.). Paris:Bailliere, 1839–1861.

Hippocrates. *Complete Works, with English translation.* W. H. S. Jones and E. T. Withington (Eds.). London:Heinemann, 1923–1931.

Kennaway, E. L., Cook, J. W., Hieger, I., & Mayneord, W. V. *Proceedings of the Royal Society, Series B, 111,* 455, 1932.

Müller, Johannes. Handbuch der Physiologie des Menschen für Vorlesungen. Coblenz: Holscher, 1838.

Pott, Percivall. *Chirurgical Observations Relative to the Cataract, the Polypus of the Nose, the Cancer of the Scrotum, etc.* London: Carnegy, 1775.

Raven, R. W. Liver biopsy. *Annals of the Royal College of Surgeons of England, 56,* 89, 1975.

Rehn, L. Ueber Blastentumoren bei Fuchsinarbeitern. *Archivo klinical Chirurgia, 50,* 588, 1895.

Rous, F. P. A transmissible avian neoplasm. *Journal of Experimental Medicine, 12,* 696, 1910.

Virchow, E. I. K. *Virchow's Archiv. für pathologische Anatomie, 1,* 94, 1847.

Yamagiwa, K., & Itchikawa, K. Ueber die Künstliche Erzeugung von Karzinom. *Verhandlungen der Japanischen Pathologischen Gesellschaft, 1,* 169, 1916.

5

Ineffective Cancer Therapies: A Guide for Educating Cancer Patients and Their Families*

Daniel S. Martin, Robert L. Stolfi, and Robert C. Sawyer

Introduction

Ineffective cancer remedies sometimes are referred to as "unproven" cancer methods, "unproven" meaning that a drug has not met accepted standards for efficacy or is associated with fraudulent or quack claims. There may be, however, no deliberate intent to defraud; instead, a belief based on inadequate knowledge may be the underlying promotional incentive. The basic point of this chapter is not to distinguish between fraud and naiveté, but to demonstrate that there is a reasonable way for a layperson to recognize that a purported anticancer treatment is likely to be ineffective.

By whatever appellation, these so-called cancer remedies always have been a serious health problem and apparently will continue to be, so long as the problem of cancer remains. The despair and the desire for hope produced by cancer in its victims, their families, and their friends creates a situation in which the promise of an easy and painless treatment is difficult to resist. For the incurable cancer patient, the result is finances wasted on false hope. Even sadder is the

*The writing of this chapter was supported in part by National Cancer Institute Grant No. 1 P01 CA 25842-01A1, and the Chemotherapy Foundation, New York. This chapter was reproduced by permission of the publisher and the author, from the *Journal of Clinical Oncology* 1:154–163, 1983. Copyright © 1983 by the American Society of Clinical Oncology.

potentially curable patient who dies because a fraudulent remedy is used instead of available effective treatment.

This problem was well recognized in the early 1900s, as evidenced by President Taft's message[1] calling for consumer protection laws: "There are none so credulous as sufferers from disease. The need is urgent for legislation which will prevent the raising of false hopes of speedy cures of serious ailments by misstatement of facts as to worthless mixtures on which the sick will rely while their disease progresses unchecked." Congress responded then, and since, with laws that now require scientific proof of a drug's safety and effectiveness, with enforcement by the Food and Drug Administration (FDA). However, enforcement of these laws has proven to be difficult, as the following brief review of the most notorious of the false cancer remedies during the past 30 years reveals.

The biggest health hoax of the 1950s was the Hoxsey Herbal Tonic Treatment.[2-5] Only after 10 years of litigation were the sales of the Hoxsey Herbal Tonic Treatment stopped in the United States by a federal court injunction, and, due to legal technicalities, no penalty was imposed on Hoxsey!

In the 1960s, thousands of cancer patients eagerly sought that decade's cancer hoax, Krebiozen.[2-7] Eventually, Krebiozen was exposed as completely ineffective during an FDA court action, and public interest in Krebiozen was destroyed. Again, no penalties were levied against the promoters! One promoter voluntarily left the United States for Switzerland, where he had bank accounts, and the other continued to dispense Krebiozen under another name until he retired.

In the 1970s Laetrile[2,7-13] reigned as the major "unproven" cancer remedy despite very vigorous opposition by the FDA and many reputable cancer research groups. Although a clinical trial by the National Cancer Institute (NCI) has proven Laetrile to be ineffective as an anticancer agent,[11] it is too early to judge whether this exposé will collapse the Laetrile boom. As regards the results of legal efforts at deterrence, however, it is revealing that several key Laetrile promoters, convicted of conspiracy to smuggle Laetrile into the United States, were merely fined $10 thousand and $20 thousand, while court records revealed that one of them had banked more than $2.5 million and another $1.2 million.[12] It is not surprising that these individuals immediately returned to Laetrile promotion after their conviction.

Thus, a review of the quackery field over the last three decades makes it clear that, while the enforcement provisions of the law are available, they grind too slowly for the most effective protection of the public. And, unfortunately, there is no effective alternative movement in evidence to tighten the present legal restrictions on the promotion and sale of ineffective drugs. Since there surely will continue to be new Hoxsey's, Krebiozens, and Laetriles until the day that cancer is fully conquered, what, then, might be done to protect the public? Analysis of the promotional methods employed for cancer remedies now widely recognized as false reveals a pattern[2,14] that is common to all of them. It seems likely then, that if the public could be made aware of this promotional pattern, they would be able to identify for themselves a new unproven cancer remedy as ineffective by simple comparison and a common-sense conclusion.

In the following sections, questions aimed at illuminating the common promotional pattern of all unproven purported cancer remedies are presented with answers relevant to five ineffective remedies. These purported cancer remedies include Immunoaugmentative Therapy, or IAT[15,16]; Laetrile,[17] a chemical extracted from apricot pits and sometimes called Vitamin B_{17}; Iscador, a preparation from five kinds of mistletoe[18]; Hoxsey's Herbal Tonic Treatment[19]; and Krebiozen, a once-secret formula that turned out on chemical analysis to be only mineral oil.[20] Three of the remedies lined up for comparison in this chapter are widely accepted as proven false: one by court trial (Hoxsey), one by long-established public rejection after exposure by the FDA of lack of effectiveness (Krebiozen), and one by a definitive scientific clinical trial conducted by the National Cancer Institute (Laetrile). It is hoped that this chapter will facilitate common-sense comparison with two current purported cancer remedies and enable the lay-person to recognize that these two also belong in the same ineffective category.

Is the Treatment Based on an Unproven Theory?

The promoters of ineffective remedies explain their treatment's purported mechanism of action by using the jargon of prevailing scientific opinion. Thus camouflaged, they hope to be identified as in the mainstream of bonafide scientific thought and endeavor. To recognize this scientific "put-on," the lay-person only need ascertain whether the purported theory has been published in one of the recognized reputable scientific journals. If the proponents of ineffective cancer remedies are unable to present objective, reproducible scientific data to support their claim for drug action and for clinical effectiveness, their articles will not be acceptable for publication in the reputable scientific journals where all such publications first must undergo peer review. The latter phrase simply means that, to avoid publishing faulty or erroneous material, reputable scientific journals require review and approval by a panel of experts qualified through training and experience to evaluate the data and conclusions.

No such publications supportive of claims for efficacy are available for any of the five remedies. Thus, as discussed below, the answer to the question posed in this section is yes for all five.

IAT. Proponents claim that IAT, using allegedly specific immune human serum protein fractions, "bolsters deficient immune mechanism present in cancer victims." Although this statement roughly coincides with some prevailing immunological theories, no data ever have been offered to support these allegations, and, although the theory was announced as long ago as 1973, no report has documented it objectively in the reputable scientific literature.[15,16,21]

Laetrile. Promoters advanced two simple theories: (1) cancer cells contain an enzyme that releases cyanide from Laetrile, and the cyanide released inside a cancer cell results in the death of that cell; and (2) cancer is a vitamin-deficiency disease and Laetrile is the missing vitamin B_{17}. In reality, there is absolutely no juried evidence to support either of these theories; indeed, all published data in reputable scientific journals reveal that Laetrile has no antitumor activity against either animal or human cancers.[2,7-13,22]

Iscador. The theory advanced for this extract of mistletoe is nebulous and borders on the occult. For example, its proponents state, "In order to make an efficacious remedy . . . it is necessary to pay attention to the time of picking . . . [since the plants] not only react to the influences of the Sun and Moon, but also to those of the planets. . . ."[18] "The host tree of the plant is taken into account in selecting the form of mistletoe to be used, and selection is based on the sex of the patient and the site of the tumor. . . ."[23]

There is no objective evidence of efficacy published in the reputable scientific or medical literature. It is hard to believe that such pseudoscientific jargon persuades; nevertheless, the desperateness of the cancer patient clouds reason, and many have succumbed to the false promise of Iscador.[12,18,23-26]

Hoxsey's Herbal Tonic. This purported remedy was composed of 10 herbs, a combination said to have been learned from Hoxsey's great-grandfather, whose horse was said to have been cured of a leg cancer after grazing in a field where such plants were growing. Hoxsey claimed that ". . . a major chemical imbalance in the body causes normal cells to mutate into a cancerous form . . . [his] medicines restore the original chemical environment, checking and killing the cancerous cells." No data ever were offered to support this theory. Of course, herbal medicines are not to be denigrated in general, for, in fact, many of today's effective medicines come from herbal remedies. Nevertheless, as far as the Hoxsey concoction is concerned, no objective, scientific data ever were published to support the allegation that the Hoxsey treatment was effective against cancer.[2-6,12,19]

Krebiozen. Biological products generally are recognized as being of value in medicine; hence, to many, the simple explanation that Krebiozen was an extract of the blood of 2,000 horses inoculated with a fungus that causes "lumpy jaw" in cattle seemed compatible with their hope that an anticancer remedy was at hand. Moreover, this "drug" received undue credence and had an aura of high scientific prestige because the major sponsor was Dr. Andrew C. Ivy, then Vice-President-in-Charge of the Chicago Professional Colleges, Distinguished Professor of Physiology and Head of the Department of Clinical Science of the University of Illinois. It did not seem to matter to the believers that Dr. Ivy lacked training and experience in the cancer field or that his allegations of effectiveness were unsupported by scientific evidence or that there were no publications in the reputable scientific literature.[4-7,12,13,20]

Is There a Purported Need for Special Nutritional Support?

Throughout the ages the central importance of food to humans led to a folk tradition in which food played a role as medicine. Further, with the greater understanding of nutritional requirements and the close association of good nutrition with health, and of poor nutrition with ill health and specific diseases, the way was paved for exploitation through nutritional fads. Many people are vulnerable to exploitation in the field of nutrition because there is widespread belief that the food industry has overpurified processed foods, that certain key nutritional elements (such as vitamins) have been removed, that the so-called "naturalness" of the food is gone. Thus, a great many health food stores promote the belief that certain diets can cure cancer. They sell books on nutrition, as well as foods and appliances (juicers, atomizers, crushers, and mixers) for preparing the recipes found in these books. The recipes claim dietary cures for arthritis, eye disease, insomnia, kidney trouble, and numerous other ailments in addition to cancer.[10,14,27,28]

Against this background, it is not surprising that most purported cancer remedies call for additional special nutritional supplementation and thereby also gain the support of the health food industry and various nutritional cults. Thus, IAT advises "dietary supplements . . . [as] adjunctive therapy"[21] and Laetrile is said to require a so-called "metabolic therapy" program comprising a special diet severely restricted in meat, animal products, refined flour, refined sugar, and alcohol and including large doses of vitamins A, C, and E and pancreatic enzymes.[8,10,11,17] Proponents of Iscador claim a need for a special "lacto-vegetarian" diet, along with "curative eurythmy, a new form of movement therapy . . . [that] counteracts the deformation of organs . . . ".[24,25] The Hoxsey treatment, as a folk herbal remedy, went along with the existing food folklore. Of the five remedies chosen for discussion, only Krebiozen made neither implications nor claims for special nutritional support.

Is There a Claim for Painless, Nontoxic Treatment?

All unproven cancer remedies have been promoted as "harmless" and free of the side-effects associated with the proven, orthodox methods of cancer treatment. They also are promoted simultaneously as "alternative" treatments, the implication being that they are as effective as orthodox medical therapy for cancer. Thus, since they are "harmless," the patient is informed that the painful "cut and slash" of surgery, the "poison" of chemotherapy, and the "burn" of radiotherapy all can be avoided by taking these allegedly equally effective "alternative" forms of therapy.[10,14]

Are Claims Published Only in the Mass Media, and Not in Reputable "Peer-Review" Scientific Journals?

The purveyors of ineffective cancer remedies *must* take a mass-media publication route to make their claims because their subjective, nonscientific so-called "data" are unacceptable for publication in a reputable, "peer-review" scientific journal. Thus, in seeking to stake their claims and persuade the public to buy their product, all purveyors of ineffective remedies have mounted a crusade and continuously paraded a series of promotional claims through the mass media, including newspaper stories, advertisements, articles in popular magazines, pamphlets, radio, television, and the publications of "health" organizations.

Many people believe that claims for health products must be true or else they would not be allowed in the media. This is simply not the case. The FDA can act only against misleading drug labels. The First Amendment (freedom of speech) protects the "health hustler" from prosecution for incorrect, misleading, or false health opinions made in the mass media. The major reason that they need mass-media exposure, based on nonobjective criteria (anecdotes and testimonials), is because their purported cancer remedies simply are not effective. If they were, no crusades would be necessary, for they would receive universal acceptance and the disease would be controlled.[2,4-6,9-10,12-14]

IAT. Proponents have published articles in *Penthouse, Vogue,* and *New York* magazines, along with many newspaper stories. A CBS TV program, "60 Minutes," has given IAT national publicity and credibility. In sharp contrast, there have been no scientific publications to document their alleged claims.[14,29]

Laetrile. The articles on Laetrile in the reputable scientific literature are all negative; that is, they report that Laetrile is devoid of anticancer activity in animals or human patients. Laetrile proponents ignore these scientific reports and, relying on testimonials and anecdotes, continue to promote their "alternative" treatment in popular books (e.g., *The Fight for Laetrile, Vitamin B_{17}, Forbidden Weapon Against Cancer*), journals, advertisements, radio, TV, and their own health organizations.[5,12-14,17,29-31]

Iscador. This drug is promoted by the proponents' own publications.[24-26] The reputable scientific and clinical literature contains no verification of their clinical claims.[18]

Hoxsey's Herbal Tonic. Hoxsey promoted his treatment at naturopathic conventions and in his book, *You Don't Have to Die.* Newspaper writers and editors were paid to publish pro-Hoxsey articles, but there was no publication in reputable scientific literature.[4-6,12-14,32]

Krebiozen. This remedy was promoted in books (*A Matter of Life or Death for You or Someone You Love,* with a foreword by the U.S. Senator from Illinois), lay magazines ("Real Hope to Cure Cancer," "Big Lie Bans Cancer Drug," "Doomed To Die—They Still Live") their own publications (*Ivy Cancer News*), and newspaper stories.[4-6,12-14,32]

Are Claims for Benefit Merely Compatible with a Placebo Effect?

The main promotional gimmick is the emotional anecdotal witness and the grateful testimonial-giver. Many of these individuals are quite sincere in their belief that they have been helped by the presumed remedy, but they simply are wrong in ascribing benefit to a specific anticancer effect of the drug. To partially understand this phenomenon, it is necessary to appreciate the placebo effect. Humans are very susceptible to the power of positive suggestion, particularly when ill and desperate for hope. When given a drug by a presumed authority figure (i.e., a presumed cancer expert) with the firm promise that they now will begin to feel better, to have pain relief, to eat better, and to get well, these desperately hopeful patients frequently do just what they have been told to expect. This superficially beneficial psychological result, based on the power of suggestion and the instillation of high expectations in the patient, is called the placebo effect. The anecdote and the testimonial, with regard to the effects of drugs, are subjective beliefs, not objective evidence.[2,4-7,10,12-14,32] To determine drug efficacy reliably, only strict scientific standards should be employed; namely, adequately documented quantitative evidence of objective anticancer effects, such as a measurable decrease in tumor mass.

An FDA investigation of the testimonials and anecdotes that Hoxsey had printed on behalf of his court defense to FDA charges is revealing of the reasons why this type of subjective evidence is notoriously unreliable. In this investigation, the FDA analyzed all—some 400—cases of persons who were claimed by Hoxsey to have been cured of cancer by his treatment. The FDA demonstrated in court that the claimed cures fell into three classes.

1. In this group, patients had diagnosed themselves, or had been told that they had cancer but never had had a biopsy demonstrating they had cancer. Unless the diagnosis of cancer is confirmed by a competent pathologist's histological study of a biopsy specimen, there is no proof that the original diagnosis was correct. Nevertheless, this group of patients was treated for cancer by Hoxsey. It is, of course, easy to cure cancer when the patient never had the disease.

And, of course, the testimonial of the believing and grateful patient will be very sincere.

2. Another group of patients had well-documented cancer and had been treated for it by accepted surgical or radiation methods before consulting Hoxsey. Nevertheless, despite the apparent adequacy of the previous treatment, these patients later went to the Hoxsey Clinic fearing they had not been cured. After his treatment, Hoxsey claimed the cures as his, and his grateful patients gave him his requested testimonials. However, without proper controls, of course it is impossible to determine which treatment was responsible: the conventional, or the unconventional, or a combination of both.

3. The remaining cases were people who had cancer, had received the Hoxsey treatment, and had given a testimonial but subsequently had died of cancer (the majority) or still had cancer.

Not one case of a bonafide cure was found. As stated by Young[14] this FDA analysis of all the Hoxsey testimonials substantiates, not only the placebo effect, but "The scientific inadequacy of testimonial—anecdotal evidence, no matter how sincere the testimony!" More recently,[14] the same findings were obtained in the National Cancer Institute's evaluation of Laetrile cases.[2-10,12-14,31,32]

Are the Major Proponents Recognized Experts in Cancer Treatment?

Any person can claim expertise in any field; however, a bonafide expert must have appropriate credentials. Specifically, the bonafide cancer expert should be qualified by both scientific training and experience in the field of cancer research and cancer treatment. Further, the individual should be generally recognized by peers as an expert. Like people everywhere, the individual bonafide expert can be wrong; hence, an individual expert's opinion should find concurrence with that of most other bonafide experts, before that opinion can receive the designation of "general recognition," that is, the consensus of expert opinion.[2]

The layperson who is concerned over someone's claim of expertise need only to go to a good library where published data (e.g., in the *Directory of Medical Specialists,* the *Directory of the American Federation of Clinical Oncologic Societies,* the *Directory of the American Association for Cancer Research,* and the *Directory of the American Association of Clinical Oncology*) may be found indicating that an individual has both recognition and special training and experience in the fields of cancer research and cancer treatment. As noted later, in the field of "unproven" cancer remedies, it is extremely rare to find a promoter with any credentials even remotely suggesting recognition, training, and experience.

IAT. The key promoter is a zoologist without any training either in medicine, in cancer research, or in treating cancer patients.[18]

Laetrile. The key promoters have backgrounds as follows: One is neither a scientist nor physician and has had a conviction for stock fraud. Another is neither a scientist nor a physician and represents himself as an engineer, despite never having received a degree. A third poses as a biochemist and sometimes as a physician, but has neither degree. Another is a physician but has neither scientific training nor experience in cancer research and treatment and has had his M.D. license removed for malpractice.[10,14,33]

Iscador. The leading Iscador peddlers are physicians, but none has general recognition as an expert in the field of either cancer research or cancer treatment.[18]

Hoxsey's Herbal Tonic. Harry Hoxsey had no scientific degrees and was a so-called naturopath.[4-6,19]

Krebiozen. The leading Krebiozen promoter, Dr. Andrew Ivy, was a physician and scientist with impressive credentials, but only in the field of physiology. He had no training in either cancer research or cancer treatment. Dr. Ivy was a famous physiologist who had strayed from his field of competency. He may have had good intentions and been misled by his lack of knowledge of the cancer field—or he may have been a fraud. Regardless, his opinion should not have been accepted blindly.[4-6,20]

Do Proponents Claim Benefit for Use with Proven Methods of Cancer Treatment? For Prolongation of Life? For Use as a Cancer Preventive?

All of these three claims for benefit require concomitantly conducted, randomized control groups of cancer patients for experimental evidence. This never has been done by the purveyors of unproven methods of cancer treatment.

Without such experimental controls, there is no way to separate the unproven method from the concomitantly administered proven method of cancer treatment when making a claim for benefit. Without such controls, prolongation of life is merely a "guesstimate" that the patient is living longer than someone expected. Without such controls, a claim for cancer prevention is somebody's belief that the patient would have developed cancer were it not for the presumed action of the unproven drug. Nobody can predict accurately either the survival time of an individual patient or which person will develop cancer.[2] Nevertheless, the purveyors of unproven cancer remedies claim these benefits without the objective evidence of a comparable nontreated control group. The underlying reasons for this failure seem obvious. Objective data would present a sharp contrast and rebuttal to placebo claims. Explanations for this lack of objective data all plead a common promotional refrain. In the 1950s, Hoxsey claimed he was " . . . kept too busy to spare the time, personnel, and facilities for objective study."[2] Today's promoter of Laetrile states, "We have neither the time nor the personnel to be a research institute. We are too busy treating patients."[34]

Yet, disturbingly, such promoters do claim excellent anticancer treatment results and have been shown in court actions to have collected millions of dollars on the basis of these claims. Surely, if they lack the time or scientific training or research background to gather objective data themselves to judge the true merit of the method they are promoting, they have the funds to engage competent research personnel to do this important task for them. Ethical pharmaceutical concerns do this all the time. There is no excuse for anyone being unaware of the strict criteria for scientific investigation necessary before a drug or treatment method is acceptable for medical use, and these promoters certainly have the means (money, patient volume, and facilities) to gather the requisite objective data.

Is There a Claim That Only Specially Trained Physicians Can Produce Results with Their Drug, or is the Method of Drug Preparation Secret and Available Only from them?

IAT. The precise details of the method of biological preparation are kept secret; therefore, only the promoters can make it for distribution.[15,16,21] And, since there are no details published of their secret methodology, no reputable scientist can repeat, and thereby either confirm or refute, their claims of alleged benefits.

Laetrile. Promoters state that one " . . . cannot expect to get results from Laetrile treatment unless you are a trained metabolic physician."[2] Translated, this essentially means that the particular physician must be a Laetrile proponent to begin with.

Iscador. Proponents state that the physician must be an "experienced anthroposophical practitioner," that is, trained to administer mistletoe therapy, and "to see man again as a whole being, consisting of body, soul and spirit." The proponents state that the " . . . difficulty is in finding . . . enough doctors trained in its therapy."[18,24-26]

Hoxsey's Herbal Tonic. Hoxsey's herbal prescription was available only at a Hoxsey Clinic, and the bottle states, "Not refillable except . . . in Drug Dispensary of Hoxsey Cancer Clinic."[5]

Krebiozen. This was a secret prescription, available only from the Krebiozen Research Foundation, and turned out to be mineral oil.[4-7,20]

Is There an Attack on the Medical and Scientific Establishment?

A favorite gambit of all promoters has been the charge that the scientific, medical, government, and pharmaceutical "establishment" are in a conspiracy to prevent a cure for cancer. They argue that doctors maintain a lucrative practice by treating cancer patients and that drug companies make enormous profits by selling worthless cancer drugs. They state that the medical establishment resists a cure for cancer because it would put an end to this economic monopoly.

The ploy is cunning, as it always is difficult to prove that something is not taking place secretly. And, if a scientific evaluation of unproven remedies is made and the result is reported as negative, proponents can and do claim that the reason is that the establishment is biased due to a greedy desire to protect the profits it makes from cancer.

A little common-sense reflection, however, will reveal that this medical conspiracy charge is not tenable. There are many other diseases that also have been "profitable," but medical scientists were not inhibited from finding vaccines for polio, insulin for diabetes, and miracle drugs like cortisone and penicillin. In the light of these facts, why would the establishment select cancer as a disease for which to prevent a cure? Doctors and their families all get cancer; why would they forgo finding a cure? Further, for an American conspiracy to work, the rest of the world's establishment also would have to be included. Could such a conspiracy cover the world, remain a secret, and have so many people forgo a cancer cure for financial greed? Further, this charge is incompatible with the fact that some other nations where there is no private enterprise and therefore no profit motive, and where large sums and much governmental effort are poured into cancer research, also have rejected these purported cures as ineffective?

IAT. Proponents state that IAT could " . . . overturn the present methods of treating cancer and render obsolete . . . the economic support of the cancer industry. . . ."[29]

Laetrile. Proponents claim that " . . . the cancer portion of the medical monopoly, enshrined in establishment orthodoxy and funded by major pharmaceutical interests, had effectively blocked the channels of information. . . . "[35] They describe the NCI negative clinical findings on Laetrile as "calculated to undermine the whole Laetrile movement."[36]

Iscador. At their meetings, their physician–proponents call for "freedom of action for the medical profession."[26]

Hoxsey's Herbal Tonic. Hoxsey termed medical specialists "rats" and spoke against the medical profession in an address entitled, "Who Are the Real Cancer Quacks and May God Have Mercy on Their Souls."[32]

Krebiozen. Proponents staged demonstrations and "sit-ins" at the offices of the FDA, claiming the scientific establishment was suppressing the use of a drug that could save lives.[4-6]

Is There a Demand by Promoters for "Freedom of Choice" Regarding Drugs?

Insistence on reliable scientific standards of objectivity for proof of drug efficacy has led to the demand for "freedom of choice" by the purveyors of ineffective cancer remedies. Since "freedom" is such a revered word in this country, they argue that the freedom to buy whatever remedies a cancer sufferer wishes is a basic American and Constitutional right. Their reason, of course, is obvious. Their ploy is to do away with consumer protection, which legally requires proof of efficacy. They want the legal freedom to defraud by misrepresentation of facts in drug labeling and selling. *Caveat emptor*—"let the buyer beware"—is an immoral, unethical, and particularly reprehensible doctrine in the medical marketplace where human life is at stake.

IAT. Proponents seek a bill in the state of Florida[37] and in Congress for freedom to use IAT without having to prove effectiveness.

Laetrile. Proponents call for a freedom-of-choice bill to remove the efficacy clause of the Food, Drug and Cosmetic Act.[2,10,14]

Iscador. Their call for "freedom of action for the medical profession"[26] may be viewed as another way of demanding "freedom of choice" in therapy.

Hoxsey's Herbal Tonic. Hoxsey said that the people's right to pick the treatment of their choice was being suppressed by a villainous and greedy conspiracy.[32]

Krebiozen. Proponents such as the National Health Federation stated that the FDA is "a ruthless enemy" of the people, one that prevents "freedom."[14]

Conclusion

The subject of "unproven" cancer remedies is a serious one, involving ethics, science, and a commitment to humanism. This chapter constitutes an endeavor to develop an educational mechanism for effectively communicating knowledge to the public that will enable citizens to distinguish the rational from the irrational in cancer treatment.

References

1. Message from President Taft. *Congressional Record* 62 Cong, 1 Sess, 2380 (June 21) 1911.
2. Food and Drug Administration: Laetrile: Commissioner's decision on status. *Federal Register* 42(151):39768–39806 (Aug 5) 1977.
3. Young JH: The medical messiahs. Princeton, NJ, Princeton University Press, 1967.

4. Janssen WF: The cancer "cures": A challenge to rational therapeutics. *Analytical Chem* 50(2):197A–202A, 1978.
5. Janssen WF: Cancer quackery: Past and present. *FDA Consumer,* July–August, 1977.
6. Janssen WF: Cancer quackery—the past in the present. *Sem Oncol* 6(4): 526–536, 1979.
7. Fischer DS: Unproven methods of cancer management, in Fischer DS, Marsh JC (eds): *Cancer Therapy for the Eighties.* Boston, GK Hall Co, in press.
8. Laetrile: The political success of a scientific failure. *Consumer Reports* 42:444–447, 1977.
9. Martin DS: Laetrile—a dangerous drug. *Ca* 27:301–304, 1977.
10. Martin DS: An overview of unconventional (fraudulent) treatments of cancer, in Aisner J, Chang P (eds), *Cancer Treatment Research.* The Hague, Boston, London, Martinius Nijhoff, 1980.
11. Study says laetrile is not effective as cancer cure. *New York Times,* May 1, 1981.
12. Wood GC, Presley BM: The cruelest killers: An update, in Barrett S (ed), *The Health Robbers.* Philadelphia, GF Stickly Co, 1980.
13. Arje SL, Smith LV: The cruelest killers, in Barrett S, Knight G (eds), *The Health Robbers.* Philadelphia, GF Stickly Co, 1976.
14. Young JH: Laetrile in historical perspective, in Markle GE, Peterson JC (eds): *Politics, Science and Cancer: The Laetrile Phenomenon.* Boulder, Col, American Association for the Advancement of Science, Westview Press, 1980, pp 11–59.
15. American Cancer Society: Cancer Immunology. New York, Immunology Research Center, Immunology Research Foundation, 1977.
16. Terry W: Summary of site visit to the Immunology Researching Island, Bahamas, Jan 1978. New York, American Cancer Society, 1978.
17. American Cancer Society: Laetrile: Background information. New York, American Cancer Society, 1977.
18. American Cancer Society: Iscadore. New York, American Cancer Society, 1971.
19. American Cancer Society: Hoxsey method. New York, American Cancer Society, 1964.
20. American Cancer Society: Krebiozen and Carcalon. New York, American Cancer Society, 1971.
21. Burton L: Immuno-augmentative approach to cancer control. Pamphlet from Immunology Research Centre, Ltd at Rand Memorial Hospital, Box F-2689, Freeport, Grand Bahama Island, Bahamas. Also available from American Cancer Society, New York.
22. Stock CC, Martin DS, Sugiura K, et al: Antitumor tests of amygdalin in transplantable animal tumor systems. *J Surg Oncol* 10:81–88, 1978.
23. Herbert V, Barrett S: *Vitamins and "Health" Foods: The Great American Hustle.* Philadelphia, GF Stickley Co, 1981.
24. Lyons RD: Inquiry casts doubt on Laetrile figures. *New York Times,* June 26, 1977, pp 1, 38.

25. Fellmer KE: A clinical trial of Iscador. *Brit Homoepathic J* LVII(1):43–47, 1968.

26. Society for Cancer Research: *Directions for the Use of Iscador in the Treatment of Malignant Conditions.* Arleshem, Switzerland, Research Institute Hiscia, 1978.

27. Bruch H: The allure of food cults and nutrition quackery. *J Am Diet Ass* 57:316–320, 1970.

28. Young JH: The agile role of food: Some historical reflections, in Hathcock JN, Coon J (eds), *Nutrition and Drug Interrelations.* New York, San Francisco, London, Academic Press, Inc., 1978, pp 1–18.

29. Herbert V: *Nutrition cultism. Facts and fictions.* Philadelphia, GF Stickley Co, 1980–1981.

30. Null G, Steinman L: The politics of cancer. Suppression of new cancer therapies: Dr. Lawrence Burton. *Penthouse,* July 1980, 75–76, 188–197.

31. Culbert M: *The Fight For Laetrile, Vitamin B17 Forbidden Weapon Against Cancer.* New Rochelle, NY, Arlington House, 1974.

32. Bradford RW, Culbert ML: *The Laetrile Phenomenon, Harbinger of Medical Revolution.* A Submission to the American Bar Association, Honolulu, Hawaii, Aug 1, 1980, from the Committee for Freedom of Choice in Cancer Therapy, Inc. Available from the American Cancer Society, New York.

33. Food and Drug Administration, Department of Health, Education & Welfare: Affidavit of James Harvey Young, Ph.D., in the matter of a rule-making procedure concerning Laetrile, April 11, 1977, Dockett No. 77N-0048.

34. Society for Cancer Research: *Annual Report, 1977–1978.* Arlesheim, Switzerland, Research Institute Hiscia, 1978.

35. American Cancer Society: Unproven methods of cancer management. New York, American Cancer Society, 1979.

36. *American Medical News,* July 17, 1981; *Medical World News,* July 20, 1981.

37. Society for Cancer Research: *Annual Report, 1978–1979.* Arlesheim, Switzerland, Research Institute Hiscia, 1979.

6

The Social and Economic Costs of Cancer

Faye W. McNaull

Cancer is a group of acute and chronic illnesses; it is fraught with exacerbations and remissions, anticipated cures and dreaded recurrences, hospitalizations and discharges, progressive and invasive treatment regimens, and, in general, a physiological and psychosocial rollercoaster existence.

From the time they enter the health care system for diagnosis, treatment, rehabilitation, and follow-up surveillance, individual cancer patients and families spend unbelievable amounts of time and money trying to gain control of the runaway metabolic process that has caused a physiological disequilibrium.

Our quality of existence is not related to our physiological condition alone, but to a complex web of psychological responses to illness and treatment and to having a dreaded disease (Ehlke, 1978). Included are sociological repercussions, such as changes in role, withdrawal from society, and responses from relatives and friends; as well as cultural factors, such as attitudes and beliefs about "being sick," "unclean," or "helpless" (Sontag, 1977). Moreover, in American society, our perception of self-worth is closely intertwined with our economic worth in terms of earning money and paying bills or in having provided for emergencies through savings accounts and hospitalization, life, or burial insurance. Loss of these economic options represents a loss of control and reinforces feelings of helplessness and hopelessness.

If there is a "psychology of cancer," it seems to be that many cancer patients will consider as worthwhile any intervention that fosters hope of living—irregardless of the suffering or of the costs to themselves and/or their families.

The purpose of this chapter is (1) to explore some of the costs of cancer to society, to individual patients, and to families; (2) to offer suggestions to health care professionals who wish to intervene in meeting financial needs, and

(3) to describe the natural history of cancer in relation to the continuum of cancer management and to explore a prevention-oriented system of resource allocation as a means of averting catastrophic financial commitments by individuals.

Measurements of Social and Economic Costs

Health economists, focusing on the costs to society, have searched for four decades for tools to measure the costs of illness and disease in human populations. Knowledge has progressed from Dublin's discussion of *The Money Value of Man* (1946) to the report from the President's Commission on Heart Disease, Cancer and Stroke (Rice, 1965) and the Department of Health, Education and Welfare surveys of the 1960s, to the national cancer surveys conducted between 1972 and 1975 (Scotto & Chiazze, 1976). Simultaneously, Rice and colleagues (Rice, 1969; Rice & Cooper, 1967) were developing progressively more sensitive parameters for measuring the economic value of an individual to society. In 1980, Rice and Hodgson compiled an excellent overview of the costs of cancer, applying modern economic concepts to analyze differences in costs by site of occurrence.

Mortality and Morbidity

Cancer is second only to cardiovascular disease as a leading cause of death in the United States. In 1977 the age-adjusted cancer death rate was 133 deaths per 100,000 population. The morbidity burden for cancer was over 3 million persons, of which 2 million were diagnosed five or more years ago. According to present rates, cancer will affect one in four individuals and two of every three families (American Cancer Society, 1980).

Although it is the leading cause of death for children of ages three to 14, cancer is primarily a disease of middle-aged and older individuals (Rice & Hodgson, 1980). This tendency reflects the 10 to 30-year latency periods associated with carcinogenesis (Hoover, 1979) and periods of relatively weak immunocompetence in humans (Herrman, 1979).

The picture is not summarily bleak. Though cancer mortality has increased for some sites (breast, colon, pancreas, bladder, and the respiratory system), it has decreased for stomach, cervix, rectum, and uterus. With the exception of lung cancer, age-adjusted death rates have leveled off or declined since the 1950s. Primary prevention, early detection, and improving treatment modalities are beginning to have an effect on death rates (American Cancer Society, 1980).

Economic Costs to Society

Using the most recent national figures on costs of disease in the United States, those estimates for 1975, neoplasms accounted for $19 to $28 billion in medical expenses, or 8 to 9 percent total medical expenditures. Direct economic costs include prevention, diagnosis, and treatment. The large proportion is attributed to hospital and nursing home care; physician's and nursing services; drugs, medical research, and training programs; and construction of facilities. Direct costs of cancer totaled $5.3 billion in fiscal 1975. Of this, hospital care accounted for 78 percent; physician's services, 13 percent; and drugs, sundries, and nursing home care, 9 percent. The proportion spent for hospital care for cancer (78%) is much greater than that spent for hospital care for all diseases taken together (47%) (Rice & Hodgson, 1980).

Indirect costs are those due to mortality, morbidity, and disability, that is, lost output. The chronicity of cancer interferes with normal lifestyles. Strauss and Garfield (1975) have made major contributions to our understanding of the management of regimens and tasks confronting individuals with chronic diseases. Undergoing diagnosis and treatment removes persons from the workplace and enforces unforeseen expenditures. Sophisticated economic manipulations incorporate earnings, a discount rate of 6 to 10 percent, varying work-experience rates, the value of household work, life expectancy, and the value of human life in arriving at dollar amounts for indirect costs.

Using 10-percent and 6-percent discount rates, Rice estimated $1.37 billion and $1.71 billion, respectively, as indirect costs for 1975. Mortality costs were greater for males than for females. Using the 6-percent rate, the indirect cost of mortality accounted for the largest proportion of the economic costs of cancer (71%), while morbidity accounted for only 5 percent. The remaining 34 percent reflects direct costs. For all other diseases, mortality accounted for 36 percent; morbidity, 24 percent; direct costs, 40 percent (Rice & Hodgson, 1980).

In summary, the proportion of direct expenditures for hospitalization and the proportion of indirect costs due to mortality are remarkably higher for cancer than for all other diseases combined.

Economic Costs to Individuals

A third category of costs, not included in estimated economic costs of cancer but used by medical practitioners (Cromwell & Gertman, 1979; Lansky et al., 1979; and McNaull, 1978) is that of psychosocial costs. These include the financial costs of psychological, social, and cultural responses to cancer as it affects patients, families, friends, and even communities (Rice & Hodgson, 1980). Some psychosocial costs are due to disfigurement; loss of motor, bowel, bladder, and sexual function; suicide; loss of savings; relocation; divorce; family dis-integration; and child neglect and behavior problems. Cromwell and Gertman (1979) describe these as "non-economic consequences of the disease and treatment regimen."

Lansky and his colleagues described the "out-of-pocket nonmedical expenditures" associated with cancer treatment such as transportation, food, lodging, clothing, family care, and gifts for other family members. Patients' loss of pay, combined with psychosocial costs, totaled more than 25 percent of the weekly family income in a population of 70 pediatric cancer patients (Lansky et al., 1979, p. 403).

Cancer Care, Inc., a New York social service organization, reported in 1973 on 115 families who requested their assistance. Direct expenses ranged from $5,000 to $50,000; the median expenditure was approximately $20,000, over 2.5 times the 1973 median annual income of $8,000. Less than half of the families incurring over $10,000 in expenses received medical insurance payments to cover their expenditures. The impact was not limited to financial problems. General family debilitation, symptoms of confusion and insecurity in children and marked physical and psychological changes in patients were documented (Cancer Care, 1973, p. 48).

In an informal survey of 10 radiotherapy patients at Duke Medical Center, annual diagnostic and treatment costs frequently exceeded income for that year. Direct costs ranged from $2,126 to $18,000, with 80 percent of the sample having third-party coverage for 75 percent or more of the costs. The uninsured 20 percent incurred hospital/physician charges ranging from $8,000 to $20,000 for which they were personally responsible (McNaull, 1978). Psychosocial costs ranged from $60 to $20,000. These included transportation to the medical center, special food, housing for lengthy radiotherapy treatment programs, frequent follow-up visits to one or more clinics (some meeting on different days), and cost of special equipment, clothing, medications, and food supplements. Extra costs of maintaining primary caregivers in the home and for childcare were included.

Lower psychosocial costs were attributed to minimal special care or equipment needs, short-term treatment regimens, and minimal travel distances to the treatment center. These findings are consistent with the data presented by Lansky et al. (1979). It is unfortunate that, in both studies, psychosocial costs included lost income due to absence from work, exhaustion of sick leave benefits, or annual leave. These belong in the indirect cost category as described previously.

Extreme overexpenditure resulted in loss of home and sale of property, exhaustion of life savings, extreme changes in lifestyle, and forced medical indulgence due to lack of income or exhaustion of insurance benefits (McNaull, 1981).

The Patient as Consumer

Accruing Catastrophic Costs. Several sources agree that medical expenditures of 10 to 15 percent of annual income represent catastrophic costs to most families in our society (DHEW, 1971; Tucker, 1970). The scenario progresses as follows:

Unless consumers have exposed themselves to a preventive screening program that has referred them to the hospital for further diagnostic tests, most clients come to the hospital because they have noted signs or symptoms of an abnormality. The first step is a detailed interview with business office representatives to determine the individual or agency responsible for the bill and to obtain a signature guaranteeing payment. After completing further demographic details, the client may be admitted to an inpatient unit.

Some institutions require routine admission laboratory tests, x-rays, and electrocardiograms as soon as possible after admission. The billing process begins as soon as the first procedure is carried out; thereafter, the patient has no direct control over the process. Physicians initiate orders for procedures, which are billed to the patient.

Spratt (1971) describes the physician as a contractor hired by the patient-consumer. The contractor subcontracts services from the hospital, laboratory, pharmacy, and so forth. Dr. Spratt advocates a mutual patient–physician decision-making process whereby cost-effectiveness data for various diagnostic procedures or treatment interventions is given to the patient so she or he can indeed give informed consent, as required by law.

A frightening concern is that anyone who has presented himself to a hospital or clinic with an abnormality is known to be under stress and potentially in a crisis situation. The literature is replete with documentation of how our society dreads cancer; we wage battle against it at every turn (Sontag, 1977). Common myths in our society are that people with cancer must necessarily have mutilating surgery, will undergo long and difficult treatment programs, will suffer unbearable pain, will waste away, and eventually will die an undignified death (Burkhalter, 1978).

Nearly everyone is afraid of the diagnosis of cancer (Ehlke, 1978), regarding it as a death sentence. Thus, cultural and social influences cause the patient psychological stress. The diagnostic tests are exhausting, but waiting for the diagnosis is also physically and psychologically draining. Decision making and time for treatment and recovery take priority over financial concerns, as they should.

It takes energy and alertness to be an efficient customer. While this energy is diverted to treatment, recuperation, and rehabilitation, costs are accumulating in the business office computer. If their insurance is paying, few patient-consumers are sensitive to costs, unless they reach a limit. When patient-consumers receive the itemized bills or begin to pay the portions not covered by insurance, they begin to be very concerned about their irreversible financial obligation. Again, their responses vary. Some, whose personal values dictate paying their bills, will liquidate property, withdraw savings—anything to pay the bill. Others do not have resources and cannot marshal sufficient funds. The effects of these situations have been described in the literature (McNaull, 1978, 1981).

Professional Intervention. Health care professionals without an understanding of health care economics sometimes exert token gestures, such as deciding not to charge for clinic visits, giving patients clinic supplies or inexpensive equipment, or failing to enter charge slips for sterile supplies and pharmaceuticals. It would be of much more lasting value, both to the individual patient and to the institution, to refer patients to business office representatives, social workers, or third-party sponsorship representatives. Physicians and nurses should be alert to financial concerns and learn to assess these needs early in the diagnostic period. Official procedures are detailed and time consuming, and some agencies will not assist patients unless application is made prior to the initiation of diagnostic and treatment procedures. Referring patients to community agencies such as public health nursing services, American Cancer Society, and Hospice, Inc., can provide invaluable support and save out-of-pocket funds.

An Epidemiological Approach

It is interesting to examine the costs of cancer from an epidemiological viewpoint, conceptualizing cancer as a disequilibrium on the health–disease continuum and as a disease with a long prediagnostic latency period in the human body. From this perspective, we see that cancer has its own natural history.

The Prediagnostic Period. The malignant process begins long before the individual is aware of signs or symptoms and before the clinician can detect them. According to Marino (1981), a tumor will not show up on an x-ray until the number of cells has doubled 27 times. It is not palpable until it has doubled 30 times. Such a mass would measure 1 centimeter in diameter. At this point, the individual probably perceives himself as "healthy."

During this period, health care efforts must be directed toward primary prevention, which includes generalized health promotion and specific protection against disease; it includes education about nutrition, exercise, and hygiene; it focuses on high-risk, vulnerable groups, with the purpose of safeguarding individuals by reducing risk factors. Stop-smoking campaigns and immunizations are specific examples of primary prevention programs (Shamansky, 1980).

The Diagnosis and Treatment Periods. As soon as disease is diagnosable, secondary prevention begins. Early diagnosis and prompt treatment shorten the duration and severity of the illness and restore optimal function as early as possible. Screening procedures are used for early detection, while treatments to limit disability are used to stabilize a disease process. Here, the individual is formally labeled as "diseased."

The Rehabilitation Period. Tertiary prevention focuses on restoring the individual to optimal function within the constraints of any disability imposed by the disease process (Shamansky, 1980). In this period, the individual may be "cured," returning to the health end of the continuum; on the other hand, if disease persists or recurs, the patient may progress further toward the disease end of the continuum.

Death. If health care activities directed at halting the disease are ineffective, death results. This can be thought of as the final or most extreme, act on the normal progression of human growth and development.

Health Care Interventions

The American Cancer Society, a voluntary agency, focuses on (1) primary prevention by educating the public to change lifestyles that are known to increase the personal risk of contracting the disease and (2) secondary prevention by educating individuals to seek early medical evaluation for any of the "seven warning signals" (American Cancer Society, 1980).

Comprehensive Cancer Centers, hospitals, and outpatient clinics are the sites for administering cancer treatment regimens: surgery, immunotherapy, radiotherapy, chemotherapy, and some rehabilitation. Nursing homes, home care agencies, hospices, and community support groups continue the rehabilitative process. Of these, treatment centers account for the largest proportion of costs. Transferring patients to secondary care facilities or discharging them home reduces costs. Outpatient treatment is less costly than inpatient treatment, unless a third party will pay exclusively for inpatient admission, as some do.

The Social Dilemma

Heretofore, national cancer monies have been directed toward research for a cure for cancer and toward treatment and rehabilitative services, while individual costs have focused on diagnosis, treatment, and rehabilitation. This trend increases both direct costs and indirect costs, since the major interventions occur after the disease is well established in the organism.

The dilemma is whether to allocate the limited financial resources so that each individual who is known to have cancer receives optimal health care or whether to allocate monies to control known carcinogens, to change carcinogenic lifestyles, and to enforce social changes that indirectly reduce incidence or reduce risk. In the pre-Reaganomic era, national and individual resources were perceived to be unlimited. Now, given a limited amount of money for cancer, the objective may be "to do the greatest good for the greatest number of people."

With high-risk groups as the focus rather than individuals, priorities change drastically. Decision making regarding regulation of environmental pollution is illustrative of the point. The answer to the question, "Who will live and who will die?" revolves around examination of (1) scientific knowledge, (2) social parameters, (3) moral and ethical considerations, and (4) what is technologically feasible. Decision-making bodies must determine the "socially acceptable risks" in setting thresholds and standards (Samuels, 1976, p. 423).

In managing the cancer problem, the highest possible benefits may be achieved best through primary prevention and early detection (Eddy, 1981). The costs of cancer to society may be reduced effectively through primary prevention; however, to sell such an idea in a treatment- and disease-oriented health care system is formidable at best.

For individuals, Reaganomics will increase financial stresses. Already we know that Medicaid payments will be reduced both for in- and outpatient care and for pharmaceutical prescriptions. Also, one must not disregard the need for catastrophic insurance coverage.

Future Trends

Future costs of cancer depend on incidence, mortality, and survival rates; on whether we focus on primary or secondary prevention; on economic trends that affect individual earnings; and on age and size of future populations (Rice & Hodgson, 1980). Regarding the latter, we know that the population is aging; therefore, given present trends, we expect rates of cancer to rise.

Future economic costs of cancer depend on the extent of cancer illness and the degree to which technology continues to inundate the medical business scene; they depend on the treatment options; and they depend on the extent to which paying patients subsidize research. They also depend on consumers: their level of knowledge, their assertiveness in making the decision to control their lives and deaths through setting limits on their own participation in a runaway process that can be financially devastating and potentially dehumanizing to them and to their families and friends.

Summary

We have painted a bleak picture of cancer costs to society and to individuals. We have illustrated the difficulties and lack of control among cancer patients and their families in "buying" services they can't afford. We have proposed the concept of primary, secondary, and tertiary levels of care superimposed on the health-disease continuum and on the periods of the natural progression of cancer. We have suggested some interventions.

The task is complex and multifaceted and may revolve around the American health care consumer's decision to exert personal and political influence on a health care system that is not accessible and is not acceptable for meeting needs because it is too costly.

References

American Cancer Society. *Cancer facts and figures: 1980.* New York: American Cancer Society, 1980.

Burkhalter, P. K. Sociocultural aspects of cancer. In P. Burkhalter and D. Donley (Eds.), *Dynamics of oncology nursing.* New York: McGraw-Hill, 1978.

Cancer Care, Inc. *The impact, costs and consequences of catastrophic illness on patients and families.* New York: Cancer Care, Inc., and the National Cancer Foundation, Inc., 1973.

Cromwell, J., & Gertman, P. The cost of cancer. *The Laryngoscope,* 1979, *89,* 393–409.

Department of Health, Education and Welfare. *Catastrophic illness and costs: Progressive analysis.* Washington, D.C.: Department of Health, Education and Welfare, 1971.

Dublin, L. I., & Lotka, A. J. *The money value of man* (rev. ed.). New York: Ronald Press, 1946.

Eddy, D. M. The economics of cancer prevention and detection: Getting more for less. *Cancer,* 1981, *47,* 1200–1209.

Ehlke, G. A. The psychological aspects of cancer. In P. Burkhalter and D. Donley (Eds.), *Dynamics of oncology nursing.* New York: McGraw-Hill, 1978.

Herrmann, C. S. Immunology: The method to our madness. *Cancer Nursing,* 1979, *2,* 359–363.

Hoover, R. Environmental cancer. *Annals of the New York Academy of Science,* 1979, *329,* 50–60.

Lansky, S. B., Cairns, N. U., Clark, G. M., Lowman, J., Miller, L., & Trueworthy, R. Childhood cancer—nonmedical costs of the illness. *Cancer,* 1979, *43,* 402–408.

McNaull, F. W. The cancer patient's financial concerns—an element in assessing nursing interventions. *Oncology Nursing Forum,* Winter–Spring 1978, 1–2, 4.

McNaull, F. W. The costs of cancer: A challenge to health care providers. *Cancer Nursing,* June 1981, 207–212.

Marino, L. B. *Cancer nursing.* St. Louis: C.V. Mosby, 1981.

Rice, D. P. Economic costs of cardiovascular disease and cancer, 1962. In *U.S. President's Commission on Heart Disease, Cancer and Stroke Report.* Washington, D.C.: U.S. Government Printing Office, 1965.

Rice, D. P. Measurement and application of illness costs. *Public Health Reports*, 1969, *84*, 95–101.

Rice, D. P., & Cooper, B. S. The economic value of human life. *American Journal of Public Health*, 1967, *57*, 1954–1966.

Rice, D. P., & Hodgson, T. A. Social and economic implications of cancer in the United States of America. *World Health Statistics Quarterly*, 1980, *33*(1), 56–100.

Samuels, S. Determination of cancer risk in a democracy. *Annals of New York Academy of Science*, 1976, *271*, 421–430.

Scotto, J., & Chiazze, L. *Third national cancer survey: Hospitalization and payments to hospitals*. Washington, D.C.: Department of Health, Education and Welfare, National Cancer Institute, 1976.

Shamansky, S. L., & Clausen, C. L. Levels of prevention: Examination of concept. *Nursing Outlook*, 1980, *28*(2), 104–108.

Sontag, S. *Illness as metaphor*. Toronto: McGraw-Hill, Ryerson, 1977.

Spratt, J. S. Cost-effectiveness in the post-treatment follow-up of cancer patients. *Journal of Surgical Oncology*, 1971, *3*, 393–400.

Strauss, A., & Garfield, C. *Chronic illness and the quality of life*. St. Louis: C.V. Mosby, 1975.

Tucker, M. A. Effect of heavy medical expenditures on low-income families. *Public Health Reports*, 1970, *85*, 419–425.

7

A Comparison of Cancer Survival Rates between Indigent and Nonindigent Populations*

John W. Berg

Economic status is related to the survival of cancer patients in several ways. Some determinants are basically social: unequal access to medical care or unequal utilization of facilities. Although such problems are important and deserving of much more consideration than they now receive, attention here will be focused on the evidence that biological differences related to economic status also have a substantial influence on prognosis.

The relation of mortality, particularly cancer mortality, to social status has been described often and well, especially for England and Wales. In these studies, however, mortality was considered a sign of differential exposure to causes of cancer, not a mark of differential response to the disease. Only in a few studies from the United States has socioeconomic status been related to survival measured from the time of diagnosis. These studies have had little impact, despite the importance of the phenomena they try to describe. This neglect reflects the complete separation between epidemiology and therapeutics. Physicians rush to report the effects of treatment on individual patients (almost never classified demographically), but ignore the impact of the same treatment on a defined population. Since epidemiologic aspects are considered so rarely in therapeutic evaluation, few physicians can be expected to sense their potential value and importance. As one consequence of this separation between

*The preparation of this chapter was supported, in part, by grant CA-15823 from the National Institutes of Health and by a gift from R. J. Reynolds Industries, Inc. to the Department of Pathology, University of Colorado Medical School.

epidemiology and clinical studies, no prospective studies on individual patients directly address the problem of exactly why people from low economic status are so vulnerable to cancer. Some speculations are obvious and will be presented at the end of this chapter. The main objective, however, will be to describe the problem as it is seen in U.S. data. The effects can be great. Indigent patients may have less than half the chance of affluent patients of being alive five years after the diagnosis of cancer. On the other hand, differences are not always that great.

It takes little imagination to think of reasons the poor of the United States might have poorer cancer survival rates. Those that are poorly integrated into the general social system could be expected to be less likely to use medical care facilities and tend to use them less efficiently. They might delay seeking medical care until their cancers were more advanced (Hackett, Cassem, & Raker, 1973, say they do; Battistella, 1971, says they do not). They may be less cooperative when treatment is prolonged, and they could be in poorer general health to begin with. It is possible that they could be receiving poorer medical care, but this would have to be documented very clearly since, in many cases, indigent care facilities are the primary resources for teaching and research and, there-fore, care would be expected to be above, not below, the national average.

Technical Considerations

At first glance, the results obtained by the half-dozen principal research groups concerned with the problem are inconsistent and the survival differences often trivial. There have been no studies planned in advance to look at this problem; all are retrospective looks at information collected for other purposes. Most re-sults could be ascribed to causes other than the biological differences we wish to consider here. But beneath these superficial differences and technical defects, I believe, lie general, pervasive, and important biological differences among pa-tients.

The first requirement for a reliable comparison of survival rates is that there be adequate numbers of patients in each group. It is no coincidence that the studies that found the link between poverty and poor survival to be consistent (regardless of the type of cancer being considered) were the studies with the largest number of patients. Much of the apparent inconsistency of results dis-appears if only groups with 60 or more patients are considered.

The second requirement, related in part to the expected large fluctuations in small numbers, is that survival differences are best seen when the group used as a standard has a moderately good survival percentage. There is little differ-ence in survival between groups when their cancers are detected and treated early, or for those with very aggressive cancers for which any five-year survival is a rarity. With such aggressive cancers, substantial differences in survival can be seen only early in the course of the disease. I have found it most useful to compare survival rates when the standard group nears 40 percent survival or when, at five years after treatment, more than 40 percent of the standard population still are alive at that time.

Third, if crude survival probabilities are the measure of the problem, age becomes an important confounding factor. The nonemployed elderly are less likely to be covered by private insurance, less likely to have other ways of paying for medical care, and less likely to live in high-rental parts of cities (area of residence has been the single most common measure of poverty in these studies). Hence, when adjustment is made for age differences, it should be invariable that fewer poor patients than affluent patients will be alive five years after their cancers are first diagnosed.

The fourth problem is the definition used to separate the poor from the remainder of the population. The most common way is to classify patients by the economic level of the census tracts (small subdivisions of a city usually containing 2,000 to 6,000 people, but varying from less than 10 to 10,000) in which they live in. Even if this were not a very indirect index of individual socioeconomic status, it still permits great variation in selection criteria. There are many choices for the economic measure: income of families or of individuals, price of house purchased, median rental, and even average level of education. Each gives a somewhat different picture of cancer incidence and survival differences. I know of no rigorous study of the reasons behind the differences that would point to one measure being more relevant than another. There also is the question of where to divide the census tracts and what groups to contrast. In an early study, Haenszel and Chiazze (1965) compared the upper and lower 35 percent of patients divided by income and found only inconsistent survival differences.

My own belief is that the effects of poverty are so concentrated in the extremely poor that it usually is necessary to look at more extreme contrasts, such as those between residents of the high and low quintiles. This, of course, has its limits, partly because the numbers can become too small but mostly because residence is such an indirect measure of poverty that one cannot achieve real segregation of the truly poor by this method. It is much better, though still far from a biologic test, to classify patients therein by current economic status. In the past, this often could be inferred from the type of hospital in which the patient was treated. The poor went to public hospitals, while the other patients chose private hospitals. This, of course, raised questions of differences in quality of care and selection by prognosis, with incurables being sent preferentially to public hospitals. There probably is no flawless indirect measure of patient status, but we must continue to seek some prognostic variable that is closely associated with poverty and is specific enough to be measured in individual patients.

Review of Published Studies

The first set of studies focusing on stage of disease and survival, as well as incidence in relation to social class, was a series of papers by Cohart in 1954 and 1955 (Cohar, 1954; 1955a,b). He found some instances of poor stage and poor survival associated with residence in lower socioeconomic areas, but felt the associations were too inconsistent to be important. Of his survival data, only those for breast cancer meet the criteria outlined previously. The five-year survival of patients from high socioeconomic areas was 48 percent, for patients in low socioeconomic areas, 38 percent.

The second study linking socioeconomic status and poor prognosis was "Morbidity from Cancer in the United States," the report of the Second National Cancer Survey (Dorn & Cutler, 1959). As shown in Table 7-1, it was found that the stage of disease varied with census tract income. Residents of the most affluent quintile of tracts had the greatest proportion of localized disease and usually the lowest proportion of disseminated disease. The differences were not very large and later it was shown (Haenszel & Chiazze, 1965) that these differences did not always result in equivalent differences in survival.

The first study reporting and discussing consistently poor survival of cancer patients appeared in 1963 (California Tumor Registry, 1963). One of the major concerns in that monograph, "Cancer Registration and Survival in Cali-

Table 7-1
Percentage Distribution of Staged Cases of White Patients,
Second National Cancer Survey, 1947

Stage:	*Localized*		*Disseminated*	
Socioeconomic Quintile: Site	*Lowest*	*Highest*	*Lowest*	*Highest*
Buccal cavity	60	64	8	6
Stomach	19	20	46	41
Colon	35	41	32	29
Rectum	43	51	25	19
Lung	24	28	43	42
Breast	43	45	17	15
Cervix uteri	51	61	13	10
Corpus uteri	56	72	16	12
Ovary	24	33	41	47
Prostate	43	52	34	34
Bladder	67	75	14	8

Source: Abstracted from Dorn & Cutler, 1959.

fornia," was the survival advantage of patients treated in private as opposed to county hospitals. This difference held for all 18 major sites tabulated, whether or not corrected for age, and for localized disease for all sites except cervix (for which survival was equal). Differences remained after correction for race and stage of disease. (This aspect was elaborated upon in 1969 by Linden without any change in conclusions.)

In 1970, Lipworth, Abelin, & Connelly sought to eliminate the problem of county versus private hospitals by considering only patients from public hospitals in Massachusetts. They divided these patients by level of income of their census tracts and found that, in general, patients from the poorer areas had poorer survival rates. They had too few patients for analysis in much detail. Only colon cancer in men and breast cancer in women met the arbitrary quantitative requirements suggested previously. In a comparison of low- versus high-income groups, three-year survival rates for colon cancer patients were 38 percent and 55 percent; for breast cancer patients, 62 percent and 71 percent. Age and stage adjustments did not change the results significantly. Unfortunately, they did not standardize by hospital or otherwise determine whether or not all of their hospitals had similar results. In 1972, Lipworth, Bennet, & Parker compared patients from public and private hospitals and confirmed the California results. At 10 months, patients from all 15 site-sex groups showed better survival in private than in public hospitals.

The National Cancer Institute published the first composite series (Axtell, Myers, & Shambaugh, 1975; Axtell, Asire, & Myers, 1977) where the stage of cancer and survival in blacks could be compared to the same statistics for whites. Blacks, almost uniformly, had more advanced disease when seen and poorer survival even with age, stage, and race adjustment. The California data had suggested that such results were partly but not completely explained by economic differences. Unfortunately, the new data did not lend themselves to economic stratification. Axtell & Myers reviewed the results in 1978, and Myers & Hankey updated the results in 1980.

In 1977, Berg, Ross, & Latourette presented a large series of cases divided by economic class but treated in the same hospital at the University of Iowa. The most important feature of the series was that, while there was a division into private and ward patients that in some cases might have been associated with different treatments, the ward patients were classified by the business office into two economic classes, even though they had been completely intermixed and indistinguishably treated in the hospital. The conclusion, confirmed by detailed unpublished case-by-case analyses, was that the survival differences between those ward patients who had health insurance and those who did not was so much greater than the difference between the insured ward patients and private patients that it was economic status and not the hypothesized treatment differences that dominated the picture. The poorer survival of indigent patients was pervasive over 39 kinds of cancer, over most stages of disease (the extremes excepted as previously noted), and at all ages from the first decade of life onward. There were enough patients with the same types of cancer that the group could be divided and the nature of the survival deficit explored in detail. Examples of the findings are presented in Tables 7-2, 7-3, and 7-4. In particular, Table 7-2 illustrates the magnitude of survival differences after adjustments for age and stage differences.

In 1980, Page & Kuntz presented a study of a large number of patients from the Veterans Administration that appears to contradict previous findings. They found no important survival differences between black and white patients (except for those with bladder cancer). Because black patients in the V.A. system in general (not necessarily cancer patients) had lower incomes than whites, it was held that their equal survival rates indicated that the results in other series were more likely due to treatment differences than to economic differences. Two alternative possibilities come to mind to explain their discordant results, although neither of them currently is supported by evidence. It may be that the income differences between blacks and whites reflected geographic differences in nominal income, rather than real differences translatable to biological differences. It also seems quite possible that the V.A. patients of all areas are biologically more alike, whatever that may mean, than the Massachu-

Table 7-2

Five-Year Relative Survival Rates[a] for Indigent and Nonindigent Patients, University of Iowa Hospital, 1940–1969

Cancer Site[b]	Indigent (%)	Nonindigent (%)
Tongue	35	48
Carotid	56	78
Other mouth	37	55
Colon	37	49
Rectum	22	43
Larynx	40	62
Melanoma	33	43
Other skin	77	96
Soft tissue	34	46
Breast	46	55
Cervix	55	64
Prostate	33	53
Bladder	34	48
Eye	57	78
Thyroid	55	74
Hodgkin's disease	29	42

[a]Corrected for normal age-, race-, and sex-specific mortality.

[b]All sites with 60 patients or more per group and over 40 percent five-year survival of nonindigent patients.

Table 7-3
Excess Deaths in First Five Years after Diagnosis of Indigent Patients,
University of Iowa Hospital[a]

Total Excess Deaths: 170/1000 patients
   Mortality: 137% of expected

Causes of Excess Deaths	Number of Patients/1000	% Excess Mortality
Older age	37	22
More advanced stage	40	24
Excess deaths due to causes other than breast cancer	32	19
General excess in breast cancer patients	20	12
Extra deaths due to indigency	12	7
Excess cancer deaths after stage adjustment	61	36

[a]Expected deaths are calculated from (1) cancer death rates of nonindigent patients and (2) noncancer deaths predicted by general U.S. rates for a population of the same sex, race, and age as nonindigent breast cancer patients.

setts or Iowa patients in public hospitals who could be subdivided into two prognostic groups.

In 1981, Berg & Finch presented data again showing some association between economic status and survival, this time for patients from Colorado cities, divided according to the income level of their census tracts. There also was a small survival disadvantage for blacks. The important point, however, was the anomalous survival behavior found for Hispanics. Members of this minority group, like blacks, were heavily concentrated in census tracts at the

Table 7-4
Excess Cancer Mortality in First Five Years after Diagnosis, Indigent Patients,
University of Iowa Hospital, with Representative Types of Cancer

Site	Excess Deaths from Cancer	Indigent Cancer Mortality as % of Cancer Mortality in Nonindigent Patients
Lip	76/1000	345
Mouth	259/1000	274
Colon	74/1000	116
Breast	101/1000	127
Cervix uteri	121/1000	152
Corpus uteri	61/1000	125

bottom of the economic scale in 1970, the time when the Third National Cancer Survey registered all cancer cases in Colorado. However, especially after adjustment for a different mixture of cancer types, the Hispanics did not show lower survival rates than those seen for Anglos (non Hispanic whites) from the most affluent areas (see Table 7-5). No reason could be suggested for the anomaly except that the Hispanics also failed to show high incidence rates for some cancers (notably lung cancer) that almost always are characteristic of poor blacks or whites.

Some Details of the Presumed Poor Survival of Indigents

Assuming for the moment that there is a group of low-socioeconomic-status patients with poor survival, it is possible to describe their survival disadvantage in some detail and even to get a rough estimate of the impact of this disadvantage in a general population. Table 7-3 describes the amount contributed by different causes to the higher death rates of Iowa's indigent patients with breast cancer. About half of the greater mortality was due to a higher death rate from breast cancer and half to higher death rates from other causes. The percentage of excess deaths in indigents ascribed to the various causes will vary from cancer site to cancer site, but the distribution given in Table 7-3 is fairly representative.

One set of stresses that we can see acting in the poor patients is their heavier burden of other diseases. Cancer patients as a general rule have greater mortality from noncancer causes than the general population of the same age, sex, and race. (This was true for 32 of 44 cancer types in one private hospital

Table 7-5
Net Five-Year Mortality from Cancer, Metropolitan Counties of Colorado

| | Anglos | | Hispanic (%) | Black (%) |
	High-income (%)	Low-income (%)		
Breast	29	33	31	41
Cervix	36	36	30	–
Prostate	34	47	38	49
Colon	51	52	41	59
All sites	49	57	55	57
Expected with site adjustment[a]	–	52	56	53

[a]Rates for high-income Anglos weighted by site distribution for each of the other groups in turn.

series; see Berg, 1965.) Indigent patients, however, have almost twice the non-cancer mortality excess of nonindigents. Linden (1969), for example, found that, for women with localized breast cancer diagnosed in California in the 1950s and followed through 1965, 41 percent of the public hospital patients had died of noncancer causes compared to only 23 percent of the private hospital patients. We found that the difference in noncancer mortality persisted as long as we could follow patients in Iowa and Colorado.

It seems self-evident that poor cancer patients would have higher general death rates than affluent patients. What is not so obvious is that they also would have excessive cancer mortality. The excess again varies by site. At times it seems more important in absolute terms, at times in relative terms (Table 7-4). In the Iowa study these excess deaths usually were not seen in patients with early cancer or in those presenting with advanced disease. In both of these groups indigent and nonindigent patients had about the same chances of dying or not dying from their cancers. It was in the patients with intermediate stages of disease, roughly those with a 30- to 70-percent chance of being cured if they were nonindigent, that the important differences in cancer mortality were seen. Among the indigent patients were some who, instead of having the expected one or two years free of disease after primary treatment before cancer recurred, developed widespread recurrent disease almost immediately and died rapidly. Such a clinical course should have implied cancer that was histologically anaplastic and agressive, yet in a small but completely matched series (indigent and nonindigent breast cancer patients matched for age, histological type of cancer, size of cancer, number of positive axilliary nodes, and treatment), I could find no histological differences in grade or in host reaction around the tumor or in lymph nodes that would explain the different course of disease in the indigents.

In the California, Massachusetts, and Colorado studies, the excess cancer mortality occurred almost entirely in the first year after diagnosis. Table 7-6 illustrates this with Colorado data. The observed cancer mortality for the patients from poor areas is compared with expected values (the rates found for patients from the most affluent areas, adjusted to the site distribution found in patients from poor areas, who usually have more aggressive types of cancer; see Berg & Connelly, 1979). As is evident, after an appreciable excess cancer mortality rate in the first year, the rates for the next seven years (about the same cumulative rate as in the first year) were equal in the two patient categories. The first year's data, also presented month by month, show the absolute differences are greatest in the first few months, as emphasized by Lipworth, Bennett, & Parker in 1972, but large relative differences persist for the entire 12 months, at least in these data.

The Iowa study gave different results, in that excess cancer mortality continued to be seen for many types of cancer after the first year. Table 7-7 contrasts the findings in the Iowa and Colorado series on a site-by-site basis. The reason the data and discrepancies are presented in detail is that it seems of

Table 7-6
Cancer-specific Mortality Rates for All of Colorado: Low Socioeconomic Strata Patients[a] Compared to Site-adjusted Rates from High Socioeconomic Strata Patients[b]

Time after Diagnosis	Observed (low-income)	Expected (adjusted high-income)	Ratio
1st month	.090	.061	1.481
2nd month	.076	.061	1.241
3rd month	.053	.043	1.246
4th month	.041	.038	1.077
5th month	.033	.035	0.946
6th month	.032	.033	0.979
7th month	.026	.021	1.218
8th month	.034	.026	1.332
9th month	.025	.026	0.959
10th month	.023	.014	1.705
11th month	.022	.019	1.143
12th month	.015	.009	1.623
1st year	.383	.325	1.179
2nd to 8th year	.348	.350	0.992

[a]Residents of the quintile of census tracts with the lowest median family income, 1970 census. 1969–1971 cancer cases.

[b]Residents of the quintile of tracts with the highest median family income.

Table 7-7
Number of Years after Diagnosis That the Indigent Cancer Mortality Rate Remains Substantially Higher than the Rate for "Affluent" Patients

	Iowa	Colorado
Colon	2	1
Rectum	4	1
Prostate	9	7
Lung	3	1
Breast	6	1
Bladder	3	1
Cervix	2	0
Corpus	1	2

some practical importance whether cancer susceptibility is "all or nothing," as most of the data imply, or whether it is manifested at several levels over several years after diagnosis, as the Iowa data seem to suggest. The Colorado data, for example, imply that there is a relatively small pool, 3 percent of all cancer patients, who are very vulnerable and nonresistant to cancer. Excluding this 3 percent, the remainder of indigent patients would have their cancers behave like cancers in the general population, even though the patients continued to die of other diseases at a higher than normal rate.

Another question related to cancer behavior in indigents is whether the rapid spread seen after diagnosis also can occur before diagnosis. If this were true it would mean that at least some of the advanced stage of disease characteristic of indigent patients was not due to excessive delay in seeking treatment.

The Colorado study was small in scale and could not be pursued beyond very superficial analyses, but it did offer one special opportunity: the chance to calculate the impact of the poverty factors in a total population. In the Colorado cities studied there was a population of 1,323,615 Anglos in 1970. This population developed 9,912 new cancers (excluding squamous cell and basal cell skin cancers) during the years 1969 to 1971. Among these patients, about 30 percent died of their cancer within a year. If all of these patients had had the site-specific cancer death rates found for patients living in the most affluent areas, there would have been about 9 percent fewer cancer deaths in that first year. Of course, if there were patients in the affluent areas who responded to their cancers like indigents, even more than 9 percent of the first-year deaths would be due to the "indigent factors."

By similar calculations that include adjustment of noncancer mortality for age differences, we calculated from the Colorado data that in the first five years there were 9 percent more deaths from other causes in the total population of cancer patients than would be expected from the rates of the most affluent areas. This figure is interesting not only because of the impact on cancer patients but also because of what it suggests about the impact of poverty in that general population.

Conclusions and Speculations

There seems little remaining doubt that the results of treating cancer depend to some extent on the general health of the patient. "Autonomous" though cancer cells may be, it would appear that their growth and spread, like the growth and spread of tubercule bacilli, depend in part on host vulnerability. The analogy suggests that the improving survival rates we are seeing for cancer patients may be due in part to improved economic and social factors. It also suggests that the disturbing contrasts seen after the war between survival rates in the United States, on the one hand, and in European countries on the other (Cutler, 1964) may well have lessened or disappeared. The few comparisons I have been able to make from published data suggest this is true, but there is need for another organized and concerted look at multinational treatment data. This time, however, there should be some effort to include socioeconomic variables in the presentations, not only to permit more appropriate comparisons but to indicate the importance of these factors in the different populations.

At the level of basic science, there seems to have been no study directly relating cancer susceptibility of the poor to any nutritional or immunologic deficit. On the other hand, there are a multitude of reports, far too many to summarize, linking poor prognosis to poor immune competence and the latter to poor nutrition. Hyperalimentation and immune stimulation are both receiving attention as adjuncts to direct anticancer therapy, but both seem to be producing mixed effects. Immune stimulation apparently can stimulate suppressor T cells selectively and thus actually lower host resistance to cancer. Hyperalimentation seems to reduce early deaths from treatment complications (Smale, Muller, Buzby, & Rosato, 1981) but, like immune therapy, may favor rather than impede tumor growth (see the review in Nixon, Lawson, Kutner, Ansley, Schwarz, Heymsfield, Chawla, Cartwright, & Rudman, 1981). Yet there still seems good reason to expect that as we learn more about tumor–host interactions we will learn how to strengthen the host specifically and selectively.

Another point about socioeconomic status and survival is of importance, at least in the United States. Therapeutic trials, for obvious reasons, usually are based in teaching hospitals. Many, perhaps most of these, preferentially care for indigent patients. To an undocumented extent, trials in these hospitals may involve unrepresentative numbers of nonprivate patients. For rare cancers there may be little selection bias, but for common cancers the patients in clinical trials are likely to be quite unrepresentative of the general population with the same disease. For example, in first reports from the largest U.S. breast cancer trial, five-year mortality for women aged 50 to 69 with localized disease was 25 percent (Fisher, Ravdin, Ausman, Slack, Moore, & Noer, 1968). For all women of the same age and stage of disease in the entire state of Iowa in 1969, the five-year mortality calculated in the same way was 10 percent (Berg & Robbins, 1977). The patient samples were obviously quite different, and it came as no surprise that the Iowa population showed different results from treatment. Radical mastectory gave better survival than less extensive operations and, in patients with positive axillary nodes, postoperative irradiation improved survival but only when high-voltage machines were used. Unfortunately, although these results were derived from an entire population, they do not represent randomized treatment assignments. What is needed, but is not yet achieved in cancer treatment studies, are well-designed trials in epidemiologically defined populations. Different treatments may be appropriate for different kinds of patients, and effective treatments may be discarded if they are tested on inappropriate types of patients, including those from special socioeconomic groups.

References

Axtell, L. M., Asire, A. J., & Myers, M. H. (Eds.). *Cancer patient survival.* Report No. 5, Washington, D.C.: U.S. Department of Health, Education and Welfare, 1977.

Axtell, L. M., & Myers, M. H. Contrasts in survival of black and white cancer patients, 1960–1973. *Journal of the National Cancer Institute,* 1978, *60,* 1209.

Axtell, L. M., Myers, M. H., & Shambaugh, E. M. (Eds.). *Treatment and survival patterns for black and white cancer patients, 1955–1964.* Washington, D.C.: U.S. Department of Health, Education and Welfare, 1975.

Berg, J. W. (Ed.). *Statistical report of end results, 1949–1957.* New York: Memorial Hospital for Cancer Allied Disease, 1965.

Berg, J. W., & Connelly, R. R. Economic status and cancer incidence in Colorado. In E. Grundmann & J. W. Cole (Eds.), *Cancer Centers.* Stuttgart: Gustav Fischer Verlag, 1979.

Berg, J. W., & Finch, J. L. Economic status and survival of cancer patients. In *Proceedings of the American Cancer Society's Third National Conference on Human Values and Cancer.* New York: American Cancer Society, 1981.

Berg, J. W., & Robbins, G. F. Selection of treatment regimens for women with potentially curable breast carcinoma. *American Surgeon,* 1977, *43,* 86.

Berg, J. W., Ross, R., & Latourette, H. B. Economic status and survival of cancer patients. *Cancer,* 1977, *39,* 467.

California Tumor Registry. *Cancer Registration and Survival in California.* Berkeley, Calif.: State of California Department of Public Health, 1963.

Cohart, E. M. Socioeconomic distribution of stomach cancer in New Haven. *Cancer,* 1954, *7,* 455.

Cohart, E. M. Socioeconomic distribution of cancer of the female sex organs in New Haven. *Cancer,* 1955, *8,* 34. (a)

Cohart, E. M. Socioeconomic distribution of cancer of the lung in New Haven. *Cancer,* 1955, *8,* 1126. (b)

Cutler, S. J. (Ed.). *International symposium on end results of cancer therapy.* National Cancer Institute Monograph 15. Washington, D.C.: Department of Health, Education and Welfare, 1964.

Dorn, H. F., & Cutler, S. J. *Morbidity from cancer in the United States.* Public Health Monograph 56. Washington, D.C.: U.S. Department of Health, Education and Welfare, 1959.

Fisher, B., Ravdin, R. G., Ausman, R. K., Slack, N. H., Moore, G. E., & Noer, R. J. A report upon surgical adjuvant chemotherapy in breast cancer: Results of a decade of cooperative investigation. *Annals of Surgery,* 1968, *168,* 337.

Hackett, T. P., Cassem, N. H., & Raker, J. W. Patient delay in cancer. *New England Journal of Medicine,* 1973, *289,* 14.

Haenszel, W., & Chiazze, L. Jr. Survival experience of cancer patients enumerated in morbidity surveys. *Journal of the National Cancer Institute,* 1965, *34,* 85.

Linden, G. The influence of social class in the survival of cancer patients. *American Journal of Public Health,* 1969, *59,* 267.

Lipworth, L., Abelin, T., & Connelly, R. R. Socioeconomic factors in prognosis of cancer patients. *Journal of Chronic Disease,* 1970, *23,* 105.

Lipworth, L., Bennett, R., & Parker, P. Prognosis of nonprivate cancer patients. *Journal of the National Cancer Institute,* 1972, *48,* 11.

Myers, M. H., & Hankey, B. F. *Cancer patient survival experience.* Washington, D.C.: U.S. Department of Health and Human Services, 1980.

Nixon, D. W., Lawson, D. H., Kutner, M., Ansley, J., Schwarz, M., Heymsfield, S., Chawla, R., Cartwright, T. H., & Rudman, D. Hyperalimentation of the cancer patient with protein-caloric undernutrition. *Cancer Research,* 1981, *41,* 2038.

Page, W. F. & Kuntz, A. J. Racial and socioeconomic factor in cancer survival. *Cancer,* 1980, *45,* 1029.

Smale, B. F., Muller, J. L., Buzby, G. P., & Rosato, E. F. The efficiency of nutritional assessment and support in cancer surgery. *Cancer,* 1981, *47,* 2375.

8

Treatment of Patients with Pain Due to Cancer

Benjamin L. Crue, Jr.

The problem of pain, even that related to terminal malignancy, has to some degree (like the chronic pain problem in general) been de-emphasized, or even "swept under the rug," not only by the medical profession, but by many components of our health care delivery system. The economic (as well as the individual) burden of patients with chronic pain in this country has been neglected, and it now is estimated belatedly that the cost to our national economy each year in these United States amounts to many billions of dollars. While patients with terminal cancer who have pain may be only a small fraction of this overall problem of chronic pain, they are not insignificant in total and the ramifications of their condition extend far beyond the therapeutic attempts of either the neurosurgeon or the anesthesiologist.[1] Furthermore, the suffering of each individual human so unfortunately afflicted cannot be ignored; nor can we avoid acknowledging the dread of the pain associated with terminal cancer, which has been found to be rather widespread and pervasive in our society. Indeed, it has often been proclaimed that it is not death from cancer that is feared as much as the horrible process of dying with its accompanying suffering and loss of dignity.

Definition and Classification of Pain

Communication about pain does remain difficult. We do not even have a good definition of pain. As clinicians we accept pragmatically that pain is anything that the patient says it is. Yet this acceptance of the individual patient's expression of subjective pain and suffering is not in itself entirely satisfactory, especially from an objective, scientific viewpoint, and it emphasizes the fact that we do not yet understand fully many of the underlying mechanisms involved in pain. The ongoing pain of patients with terminal cancer is incredibly complex,[2] due to the differences between etiology and mechanism and between both peripheral and central mechanisms as they relate to both acute and chronic pain syndromes. Because of the human ability to project imagination into the future, mental anguish also must be added to pain and suffering, forming a well-known, fearsome triad.[3] This initial problem of definition and the concomitant difficulty of understanding underlying causes and mechanisms leads to a confused state today, even for the classification[4,5] of human pain syndromes, and this must be discussed to some degree in this chapter before proceeding to talk specifically about pain in the cancer patient.

There is still controversy as to whether even acute pain should be considered primarily a sensation or would be better considered as a perception in relation to all human pain syndromes.[6] Pain subjectively exists only when it is felt consciously and recognized (perceived) by the patient, which leads clinically to the classification of both the discriminative and affective aspects of pain as being basically percepts. When it comes to chronic pain there can be no contesting the clinical observation that, as suffering persists over time, it seems to involve more and more central factors. In many patients with chronic benign (nonneoplastic) pain syndromes, it would appear that the pain becomes entirely central and that there may well be continued pain even in the absence of any continued nociceptive input from the original organic pathology in the periphery. There is still controversy[7] as to whether therapy in a given patient should be directed toward interrupting or altering assumed continuing peripheral nociceptive input (the "peripheralist" viewpoint), or whether all attempts at therapy (including peripheral nerve blocks, acupuncture, TENS, or biofeedback) should be done on the assumption that they have their beneficial effect (when it occurs) due to some central mechanism, (referred to, in general, as the "placebo" response).[8] In reality, treatment directed toward such a presumed central generator mechanism,[9-13] utilizing suggestion, would be a form of psychotherapy and thus is concordant with the concept of the "centralist" viewpoint. This is true particularly in that we may hope that all such therapies can be maximized consciously, or at least utilized subconsciously, for central retraining of learned perception, as well as for altering any subsequent behavioral response.[2]

Acute pain and chronic pain are usually very different, resulting in the various suffering syndromes seen in the human. Attempts have been made to classify pain as *acute, subacute, recurrent acute,* and *chronic.* This classification, however, also must include patients with *ongoing* pain due largely (or at least initially) to continued nociceptive input from untreated or untreatable peripheral pathophysiology, of which terminal malignancy is perhaps the best and most classic example. Table 8-1 represents our attempt at temporal classification of pain complaints. (In an attempt to shorten this chapter about what is, in reality, almost a limitless subject, we simply will refer here to a number of our

Table 8–1
Temporal Classification of Pain Complaints

---

1. *Acute*: May last up to a few days; mild or severe; cause known or unknown; presumed nociceptive input; emergency response; the "fix me" medical model
2. *Subacute:* May last a few days to a few months; although not an emergency, in most ways treated like acute
3. *Recurrent Acute*: Examples include arthritis (either rheumatoid or osteoarthritis), migraine, primary trigeminal neuralgia recurrent or continued nociceptive input from an underlying chronic pathological process; also may be entirely central, e.g., tic pain
4. *Ongoing Acute*: Due to uncontrolled malignant neoplastic disease (not really chronic)
5. *Chronic*: Benign (non-neoplastic) but with seemingly adequate coping by the patient; usually lasts over 6 months; no known nociceptive peripheral input; pain often made more severe by any type of subsequent sensory input; basically a "central" pain
6. *Chronic Intractable Benign Pain Syndrome (CIBPS)*: Chronic pain with poor patient coping

---

articles published on this subject; the reader is encouraged to use the references to direct further study.)

Pain in Cancer

It is unfortunate that pain in cancer patients usually serves no useful purpose. It also is unfortunate that pain is only very rarely an early warning sign in the development of any type of malignancy, in almost any location. Instead, pain in patients with malignancy is often a late sign, seen in the terminal aspects of the condition, and may be truly severe only very late in the disease process. The pain may occur even long after attempts at surgical removal, irradiation therapy, chemotherapy, and immunotherapy have been tried and, although sometimes palliative, have been proved largely ineffective. This reminds us of the couplet that often is heard from our colleagues, who may at times deride those who have an interest in trying to alleviate or ameliorate the pain and suffering of these unfortunate individuals: "Things are looking mighty grim/The neurosurgeon has been called in." Unfortunately, such sentiments usually reflect only the speakers' prejudices and lack of understanding of the treatment of pain (the specialty of "algology"), even by many members of the medical profession. The claim made here is that we understand more about the pain in patients with underlying cancer and often are more successful in the therapeutic treatment of pain due to cancer than we are in many other pain syndromes. Certainly the treatment of a patient with cancer pain that is due to continuing nociceptive input is far easier, from both a technical viewpoint and an understanding of the underlying etiology and mechanism, than treatment of those with the so-called chronic benign (noncancer) pain syndromes. The results reflect this, although of course we refer only to the relief of pain and suffering and not to the treatment of the underlying malignancy.

It would appear that the ongoing pain in patients with uncontrolled malignancy, from both an etiological and mechanistic (both neurological and psychodynamic) viewpoint, may require consideration of at least three major components of the suffering process: (1) continued nociceptive input, (2) central psychological mechanisms, and (3) threat of impending death.

Continued Nociceptive Input

The majority of patients with cancer will have some pain and at some time it will be of clinically significant severity.[14] This aspect of acute (nociceptive input) pain from the ongoing malignancy usually plays the leading role in the dying cancer patient's suffering. There is almost always at least some significant element of ongoing acute organic pain due to underlying cancer, where the malignancy is advancing in spite of all attempts at therapy. The most common reasons for pain due to tumor invasion, regardless of the type of malignancy, are the compression or invasion of the perineurium of major nerves (often the brachial or lumbosacral plexus), and bony metastases (with or without pathological fracture).[15] This known organic peripheral etiology, as well as the underlying presumed peripheral mechanism for the initiation of nociceptive input into the peripheral nerves to be carried to the central nervous system centripetally, justifies the concept and the assumption that there is continued peripheral nociceptive afferent input. This input, however, often can be blocked successfully by anesthesiological or neurosurgical procedures to interrupt the sensory input pathways. The decrease of suffering after successful surgical or anesthesiological nerve block attempts may be accompanied not only by amelioration of the suffering but an actual increase in the quality of the patient's survival and, on occasion, a demonstrable increase in the patient's survival time.

Most articles on neurosurgical treatment of pain include lists of the state-of-the-art (plus newer investigational or experimental) techniques to attempt to interrupt this nociceptive input in patients with ongoing cancer pain. The interested reader is referred to standard works on neurosurgical pain relief procedures or anesthesiological nerve block techniques, as well as to a few procedures relative to our own particular interests along this line.[16-30] It should be pointed out that in discussing results reported from therapeutic attempts at pain relief, regardless of what pain syndrome one is talking about, the following five points always should be considered:

1. Patient selection
2. Goals of therapy
3. Specific modalities of treatment

4. Immediate results
5. Long-term results and recidivism rates

Patient Selection. When conducting any study, one must take care not to compare apples with oranges. For example, if the author is writing an article on percutaneous chordotomy, it must be made clear to the reader that the author probably is *selecting* only patients with unilateral pain, as bilateral or paravertebral pain in terminal malignancy is much more difficult to treat. It is true that presently the most common tumor in the male is cancer of the lung and in the female cancer of the breast; most of these tumors metastasize first to the region of the brachial plexus and cause unilateral upper extremity pain. It also must be remembered that, when considering tumors common to both sexes, the most frequent is still carcinoma of the large bowel. Cancer of the colon may well have multiple metastases and, when not confined to the liver, may occur in the presacral region. This cancer usually gives bilateral pain that is not well treated by chordotomy. Thus, even in patients with cancer pain, selection is very important in the assessment of the results of treatment.

Goals of Therapy. In considering what goals were set, one must remember that it is very difficult to talk about excellent, or even good, results in terminal cancer. When doing stereotactic procedures in human beings suffering in the terminal stages of cancer, we are not treating the underlying malignancy, but are trying only to give palliation for the usually short time that is left. Furthermore, would it be an acceptable goal in, for example, percutaneous chordotomy, to relieve all pain or only to decrease the severity to where the patient will be more comfortable but perhaps even need continued narcotics? Should we accept a certain percentage of postoperative hemiparesis after percutaneous chordotomy and still consider it a good result, provided there is pain relief? These examples show how treatment goals must be understood in each case before evaluating results.

Specific Modalities of Treatment and Short- and Long-Term Results. Most reports on the treatment of cancer pain from neurosurgeons and anesthesiologists dwell on the various modalities of therapy. This is well and good, but, when it comes to talking about the results from the various modalities of treatment, we must know if the author is reporting immediate results or long-range results.[31,32] Most surgeons are as guilty in talking about immediate postoperative results in cancer pain as other authors are in talking about the results of acupuncture, transcutaneous electrical stimulation,[33] or even biofeedback in patients with chronic benign pain syndromes, where long-term results usually would demonstrate an increasing recidivism rate. Reports of good short-term results often lend an unjustified credence to the concept that such modalities are really effective. Instead, long-range results suggest that they all are probably only a form of placebo; that is, while they work through an organic central mechanism involving the endorphin system,[34] they really are forms of "suggestion leading to decreased anxiety."[8]

The same criticism can be true in writing about cancer pain. Does the author talk only about her immediate results, or is she discussing long-range results? Again, this must be viewed in light of the goals, as some authors believe that such percutaneous procedures should be carried out in the early stages of the disease where, if successful, they may well increase the quality of life for a longer period of time. The present author, however, believes that present medications for treating nociceptive input pain are effective enough (with small-enough unwanted side-effects), while most percutaneous pain relief procedures (such as stereotactic percutaneous high cervical chordotomy) carry enough risk of complication and enough decrease of good results, plus an increase in pain with a rising recidivism rate over time, that chordotomy should be carried out only in the terminal or preterminal stage of the cancer patient's illness. Therefore, if one does such operations only in the late stages, there will be no long-term results, so the important results are whether or not the pain relief from the surgery persisted and was adequate to give significant amelioration from the suffering, up to the time of death.

Central Psychological Mechanisms

The individual patient with his particular specific malignancy and his related pain syndrome also must be regarded as having both a unique perceptual experience of his pain and a unique behavioral response. Some patients with cancer pain appear to be accepting and even stoical. A few patients with cancer even seem to use the mental mechanism of denial relatively successfully to react to their cancer and even their cancer pain problem. Others seem to use quite different mental defense mechanisms and psychodynamics, many of which we can only assume are largely due to their premorbid personality characteristics. The behavioral expressions related to these internal states can be understood to some extent only if we become aware of salient points in the patient's life history. Subsequent to the development of the malignancy and its pain, these unconscious mental mechanisms become significantly involved, along with important internal reactive elements and important environmental operant factors, in a manner similar to those inpatients with chronic intractable benign (non-neoplastic) pain syndromes.[35-37] At least clinical experience has shown that there can be no contesting the fact that the individual verbal and behavioral responses to the pain suffered by many patients with advancing cancer appear in many ways to be similar—and involve identical psychodynamic mechanisms—to those seen in patients with chronic intractable benign pain syndromes.[38-40] Thus, it behooves us to take the time in this chapter to list some of the characteristics of the chronic intractable benign pain syndrome (CIBPS). This syndrome has been defined[32,39] as an ongoing problem with pain that (1) cannot be shown to be related closely in the here and now with any active pathoanatomic or pathophysiological process, (2) has an antecedent history of generally ineffective medical and surgical intervention for the pain problem, and (3) has come to be accompanied by disturbed psychosocial functioning that includes complaining and a host of epiphenomena that accompany it.

The epiphenomena common to CIBPS include:

1. Mood and affect changes that are in themselves significantly dysphoric
2. Drug dependency or abuse, of varying severity, with its attendant CNS side-effects
3. Multiple surgeries or pharmacologic treatments separate from the drug dependency issue, with their own morbid side-effects
4. Escalating psychosocial withdrawal, with increased loss of gratification from these interactional inputs
5. Interpersonal conflict with significant others
6. Increasing hopelessness and helplessness as increasing dysphoria does not give way in the face of mounting numbers of "new" or different therapies
7. Decrease in feelings of self-esteem, self-worth, and self-confidence
8. Decreasing ability to obtain pleasure from the life process, contributing to profound demoralization and, at times, significant anhedonia, if not depression
9. Escalating physical incapacity, partly due to inactivity because of fear of increasing pain discomfort or of causing more bodily harm; fear based on the belief that ongoing pain is a signal of increasing bodily damage
10. Conflicts with medical personnel (doctors, nurses, therapists, technicians), with resulting dissatisfactions and/or hostilities

It has been our observation that many of the patients with cancer pain and suffering over the years have demonstrated all of these problems. They are not usually sequential, as outlined by Kübler-Ross[41]; rather, they occur in various combinations and to various degrees, and ambivalent or contradictory feelings and behaviors can and do occur concomitantly as well as sequentially in the terminal patient with cancer pain.

Over the years, a significant number of patients in our CIBPS unit[42] who apparently have undergone previous successful treatment of their underlying malignancy have continued to have chronic pain, usually in the region of their previous cancer or surgical operation or radiation site. Often this pain has continued for years after all evidence of any residual tumor, or even where concern on the physician's part over probable recurrent malignant neoplasm was no longer a significant realistic medical consideration. These "cured" cancer patients had a true CIBPS. Here the experience of having had the cancer (and the concern, conscious or unconscious, of the possibility of recurrence, or of another cancer) becomes one of the psychodynamic mechanisms in the development of the CIBPS, as there is no evidence for any continued nociceptive input, including none from "the scar," which appears to be identical in these patients with scars in other cured patients who have no continuing pain syndrome. This is usually accompanied by a state of ongoing fearfulness that may present itself as a serious hypochondriasis or a chronic generalized anxiety with features of depression. Depression itself may episodically become the major observable problem. At times a frank cancer phobia may emerge. However, the main central complaint of the patient remains unrelenting pain. Associated with this are strong overt or covert cognitive links on the patient's part between the pain and old or fresh revisitations of cancer. This in form is very similar to the patient with CIBPS who has been through multiple surgical procedures for a pain problem that has not relented. Many of these patients continue to believe firmly that the continuing experience of pain can be related only to present and ongoing pathology.

Thus, in chronic pain related to cancer, there may be overlap both ways. Patients with pain due to cancer may have psychodynamic mechanisms similar to the CIBPS patient, while a number of the patients with CIBPS may have, as part of their dynamics, a justifiable fear and anxiety concerning the possibility of underlying malignant disease due to their past experience of cancer in themselves, their family members, or close friends.

The Threat of Impending Death

The patient with ongoing suffering and a diagnosis of causative incurable malignant cancer (whether he has been told this directly or only fears that it is not curable, being too frightened to ask or truly not wishing to know) adds a third dimension that now must be considered. The fear of impending death has been described previously by many authors such as Dolan,[42] Worcester,[43] and Oelrich.[44] The fear of dying is not unique in the cancer pain patient. It is often basically the same human fearfulness experienced by most of us, only in a more pervasive and intense threatening context in the patient with pain from terminal cancer. For example, in CIBPS, patients, especially older ones, may have considerable fear and anxiety concerning impending death, without having any underlying malignancy. Furthermore, many patients with CIBPS who have experienced an unresolved loss of health, of an extremity, of physical function, or of youth seem to have these losses or grief as part of their underlying emotional central chronic pain mechanism. This is in many ways similar to (although admittedly often less intense than) the syndrome seen in patients with pain from terminal malignancy. There is no question but that unresolved grief over loss of a bodily function and the fear of impending death are often intertwined in any patient with terminal cancer. The resulting psychodynamic mechanisms, although they may appear different, often are very similar but more intense, and are seen in a different context.

The psychotherapeutic approach to the CIBPS patient should include an attempt to uncover and understand better these unconscious psychodynamics, so that the patient can adapt better to these life forces, relieve her unjustified or justified unconscious emotional conflicts, and decrease her dysphoria and permit fuller life function. In patients with terminal malignancy, however, it often is much better to be supportive and not to attempt to be confrontational about their use of unconscious defense mechanisms in their regressed or otherwise apparently inappropriate behavior by any such psychotherapeutic attempt. This is especially the case if the defenses seem to be serving the patient well, in the sense of helping the patient to avoid temporarily some more serious mental decompensation. This is even more the case when the particular patient only has a short time to live. For example, one of the most primitive and yet powerful mental defense mechanisms is denial. Under more ordinary and less overwhelming conditions, its unconscious and extensive use might be pathologic and destructive. However, it would be unconscionable in many cases for the therapist to attempt to weaken the effect of the patient's denial in a near-terminal situation, if it is serving as a useful defense function and does not result in dysphoria in that individual patient. We must remember that terminal illness implies not much real time remaining, so mental mechanisms such as denial can be very effective and helpful for short times when a person anticipates being overwhelmed.

One often encounters unrealistic hopes in dealing with cancer pain patients. They often believe that, if only their pain could be decreased, they not only could be rehabilitated but, in fact, they would be able to get back to work, if not enter the next Olympics. They often tend to suppress or repress the seriousness of the problem causing their pain. Under these circumstances, the treator must be realistic while gently answering the patient's questions with appropriate truth and candor. While it serves no useful purpose to destroy a patient's illusions when they are working as part of a useful defense mechanism that has no real risk of crashing down in the time the patient has left, if the patient senses that you have joined her condescendingly in impossible goals, she can lose trust and faith in you as a helper. The emotional results of this can be disastrous for the patient.

As is well known to all psychotherapists, the anger and the nonacceptance of the pain, let alone the diagnosis of malignancy, is often directed outward and often toward members of the pain treatment team. The team members must be mature enough to accept this, as well as educated enough to understand it and not take it personally, knowing that the anger of the patient under such circumstances not only may be a good catharsis but also a good defense mechanism. It is far better than having the patient direct the anger inward and withdraw into depression. Unfortunately, when it is directed toward members of the patient's own family and the nonprofessional support team, it often requires gentle intervention and explanation to the family members, so as to spare their feelings and help them to accept the patient's apparently inappropriate anger.

Treatment

It is the present author's belief that the main enemy of these patients is not cancer; nor is it death, nor the pain itself. It is lonesomeness and despair. A definition of hell on earth might well encompass being elderly, sick, poor, dying, in pain, and being isolated alone, with no one who cares. Thus, over the years, it has become apparent, not only for the general well-being of the dying patient with cancer and pain but for the actual degree and severity of the pain itself, that the two most powerful factors appear to be underlying parameters over which the physician alone usually has very little control: (1) the support system that the patient has, as the pain increases and death approaches and (2) in numerous cases, the sincerity of the patient's own religious belief in a benign god and in a life hereafter.

The Support System

When it comes to talking about support, the most important thing, obviously, is the patient's own family, particularly the spouse or significant other. There really can be no truly effective substitute for a loving home environment; however, this is not always available to the patient. In fact, on some occasions, it is easier for the health care team to be a surrogate family and a support system by proxy, than to deal with a family that is not only nonsupportive but actually negative when it comes to relating to the particular patient in his or her hour of need. At times, not only does this type of less-than-optimum family situation do the patient no good and contribute to the formation of many of those psychodynamic (especially reactive) problems already discussed under chronic intractable benign pain, but it may even get in the way of the support attempted in the therapeutic milieu by the professional team.

It is here, however, that the team concept[31,45-48] comes into play. In the opinion of this author there is nothing that is as important from a therapeutic standpoint as having a truly caring, supportive team effort in the handling of these patients. This is true whether the patient is on the neurosurgical service and is about to undergo an attempted pain-relieving operative procedure, or on another pain center service where the patient may well be scheduled by anesthesiology for a nerve block, or on neurology for evaluation or for regulation of the analgesic or narcotic regimen along with antianxiety tranquilizers or antidepressants. It may be that the patient is terminal and is really at the pain center for evaluation and disposition by transfer to an extended care facility or a hospital, or to home outpatient hospice management. The members of this team are all important, and it is humbling for the neurosurgeon to realize that in many of these terminal cancer patients the degree of pain relief from his percutaneous chordotomy may be more a factor of the relationship that the patient develops with a supporting, caring paramedical team member in the hospital milieu than it is to the experience of the skill of the surgeon's technique. We have written previously about the value of the team concept[45] in the management of pain in patients with cancer, and this will not be gone into further in this chapter, except to reiterate that, in our opinion, with the passage of time, we find it more and more significant and important. To me the day is over when a neurosurgeon can see a cancer pain patient, either in his office or in an outpatient pain clinic setting within a multidisciplinary, comprehensive pain center, and then tell the patient that, since outpatient analgesics or narcotics have not worked, he should be scheduled for a pain-relieving procedure such as a rhizotomy or chordotomy the following Wednesday, and will be admitted to the hospital Tuesday for a preoperative work-up, and so forth. This is *no longer optimum and should not be acceptable medical practice.* In the first place, the patient deserves further evaluation than this. In spite of the emphasis in recent years on cost effectiveness and attempts to save money by hospital administration, medical staff, insurance carriers, and PSRO, patients with pain from cancer usually need to be evaluated in a hospital setting, with a caring pain team, before any pain-relieving surgical procedure is scheduled. It is well known that, even in a caring milieu and with family support in the home setting, narcotics often just do not have the pain-relieving effect on an outpatient basis[46] that an equal dose would have in an inpatient setting within the hospital or pain center. The patient must be admitted for evaluation and attempts must be made at conservative pain relief measures before any surgical intervention is warranted. It is true that a number of patients apparently have continued nociceptive input that cannot be sufficiently alleviated by sedation, analgesics, narcotics, anti-anxiety tranquilizers, anticonvulsants, and/or antidepressants in a reasonable dose that permits them to retain their human dignity and nearly normal mental cerebration. Moreover, anesthesiological nerve blocks and neurosurgical procedures at times definitely are indicated to cut down on the nociceptive input for pain relief. With experience, however, and with a pain team, it often is found that it is not overwhelming nociceptive input that keeps the patient's clinical pain and suffering potentiated. More frequently, it is because of uncontrollable social, economic, and psychological factors. Great care must be exercised before one should schedule an operative intervention for a cancer pain patient in the belief, hope, or reasonable expectation that cutting down on nociceptive input, or even the placebo effect of the surgical procedure itself, will have any lasting effect on pain relief. The patient's main problem may be continued pain severity due to lack of a support system or to socioeconomic or psychological problems that are beyond the pain team's control. Dr. Attila Felsööry (my late neuro-surgical colleague) and I studied our statistics at the City of Hope National Medical Center. Along with Drs. David Agnew and Jack Pinsky we developed a coordinated approach to cancer pain patients that led to the formation of a separate, distinct "pain team" concept. Over the years, we found that, although we were seeing over twice as many cancer patients with pain as five years previously, we were doing less than half as many surgical procedures and operative interventions.[49,50] Many patients with cancer pain, no matter how horrible their physical condition may seem to others, may be taken comfortably to death's door without requiring any surgical mutilation. This may be done by the judicious use of narcotics and the support of a therapeutic milieu supplied by a caring pain team.

Religious Beliefs

There is often little to be said about attempting to supply, at the eleventh hour, religious convictions to the dying cancer patient. It is not generally considered either socially or medically acceptable to attempt to proselytize to patients, regardless of their former beliefs or lack of beliefs, and regardless of what personal convictions any one member of the caring health team might hold. However, it does appear to be true that the members of the team, without exception, if they are to function effectively in this type of milieu with patients with malignancy and pain, must have at least explored the issue of their own mortality. Thus, it goes without saying that the maturity and compassion as well as the psychological stability of the pain team members' own psyche are relevant to this discussion. It is almost impossible for a treating physician, especially a surgeon, if she takes the relentless onslaught of progressive cancer to be a failure of her own previously attempted surgical operative approaches, to be either objectively or subjectively supportive to the patient under these circumstances. Both the surgeon's and the patient's unconscious feelings about death can get in the way when some physicians attempt to treat dying cancer patients who are in pain.

The usual explanation is that the specialist is too limited in time and must therefore delegate therapy (and often thereby also responsibility) to other nondoctor members of the team. This is not a satisfactory excuse, even though in recent years it has come into use not only by the surgeon but others on the team. For example, with the development of the new specialty of medical oncology, the chemotherapist can become so engrossed in the therapy of the tumor with his various chemicals that the overall treatment of the patient, let alone the handling of the patient's pain and suffering, is far from optimum. This type of observation, unfortunately, also has been found true over the years for the nondoctor members of the team, including nurses, social service workers, and psychologists. It takes time and experience to mold a truly well-functioning pain team to help care for terminal cancer patients, with or without pain, particularly within our society today, where many of the pain team members (or their spouses) are in various stages of their training, necessitating movement from one city to another and causing unavoidable replacement problems from time to time in any pain team. The problems of support for the supporters and the prevention of pain-team-member "burn-out" are also significant factors.

It also should be noted that one of the main problems that we run into repeatedly is the lack of education among pain team members concerning what is already known. For example, doctors (especially residents and interns fresh out of training) as well as nurses often do not properly utilize the tools that they have. Narcotics are notoriously underutilized medically, not only in acute pain problems (such as the postoperative recovery room or the intensive care unit) but also in the terminal cancer pain patient, where physician, nurse, and family fearfulness and moral attitudes about narcotic addiction would be ludicrous, if they were not so tragic for the individual patient. This leads to much needless suffering, as has been pointed out so eloquently by others such as nurse Margo McCaffery.[51] In addition to underutilization, there is improper use: I.M. Demerol often is used when other narcotics would be better and in doses too small and at too long intervals. Time-contingent pain medications usually are far better than pain-contingent "prn" orders. The person writing the orders must be held accountable for monitoring pain relief and for adjusting medications, doses, and time intervals appropriately. In the overwhelming majority of terminal cancer patients with pain, the gastrointestinal tract is intact. Certainly regimes such as long-acting methadone per os 10 to 40 mgm q 6 hours routinely around the clock should be tried before resorting to I.M. medications, let alone I.V. narcotics, extradural or subdural morphine, electric epidural stimulators, or experimental implanted "morphine pumps."

In conclusion, it can be stated only that, at the present time in almost all instances of patients with pain from underlying incurable malignant disease, relief of pain and suffering can be accomplished with present knowledge and present techniques. It is an unfortunate comment on our present level of medical education and training, as well as on the limitations of our health care delivery system, that such pain relief is not more universally available to these patients. Those within the system who are interested should get together and direct our efforts toward better education of health care professionals and the lay public. We must not, for example, waste time, energy, and resources in Congress attempting to legalize heroin, which appears to have absolutely no medical benefit over the already available analgesics and narcotics. It would indeed be a boon to humanity if we could concentrate our efforts where they are known to be most effective.

References

1. Kamdar M: Role of nerve blocks in the management of cancer pain, in Crue BL (ed): *Chronic Pain.* New York, Spectrum Publications, 1979.
2. Crue BL: A physiological view of the psychology of pain. *Bull Los Angeles Neurol Soc* 44:1, 1979.
3. Smith HW: Some medcolegal aspects of pain, suffering, and mental anguish in American law and culture, in Crue BL (ed): *Pain and Suffering—Selected Aspects.* Springfield, Ill, Charles C Thomas, 1970.
4. Agnew D, Crue BL, Pinsky J: A taxonomy form for diagnosis and information storage for patients with chronic pain. *Bull Los Angeles Neurol Soc* 44:84, 1979.
5. Crue BL, Pinsky, JJ, Agnew DC, et al: Taxonomy problem in pain, in Crue BL (ed): *Chronic Pain.* New York, Spectrum Publications, 1979.
6. Crue BL, Kenton B, Carregal EJA: Review: Neurophysiology of pain—peripheral aspects, in Crue BL (ed): *Chronic Pain.* New York, Spectrum Publications, 1979.
7. Crue BL, Kenton B, Carregal EJA, et al: The continuing crisis in pain research, in Crue BL (ed): *Chronic Pain.* New York, Spectrum Publications, 1979.
8. Crue BL: Some philosophical considerations of pain—suggestion, euthanasia, and free will, in Crue BL (ed): *Pain, Research and Treatment.* New York, Academic Press, 1975.
9. Crue BL, Carregal EJA: Postsynaptic repetitive neuron discharge in chronic neuralgic pain. *Adv Neurol* 4:643–649, 1974.
10. Crue BL, Carregal EJA, Todd EM: Neuralgia—discussion of central mechanisms. *Bull Los Angeles Neural Soc* 29:107–132, 1964.
11. Crue BL, Pinsky JJ: Chronic pain syndrome—four aspects of the problem, in New Hope Pain Center and Pain Research Foundation, *New Approaches to Treatment of Chronic Pain,* Research #36, Monograph Series. Bethesda, National Institute on Drug Abuse, 1981.
12. Crue BL, Shelden CH, Pudenz RH, et al: Observations on the pain and trigger mechanism in trigeminal neuralgia. *Neurology* 6:196–207, 1956.
13. Crue BL, Sutin J: Trigeminal nerve potentials and their relation to tic douloureux. *J Neurosurg* 16:477–502, 1959.
14. Foley KM: Pain syndromes in patients with cancer, in Bonica JJ, Ventafridda V (eds): *Advances in Pain Research and Therapy.* New York, Raven Press, 1979, vol 3.
15. Gilbert H, Apuzzo M, Marshall L, et al: Neoplastic epidural spinal cord compression: A current perspective. *JAMA* 240:2771, 1978.
16. Crue BL, Carregal EJA, Felsööry A: Percutaneous stereotaxic radiofrequency trigeminal tractotomy with neurophysiological recordings, in Crue BL (ed): *Pain, Research and Treatment.* New York, Academic Press, 1975.

17. Crue BL, Felsööry A: Transcutaneous high cervical "electrical chordotomy," *Minn Med J* 57:204–209, 1974.
18. Crue BL, Felsööry A: Analgesia from percutaneous periaqueductal gray electrical stimulation in the human, in Bonica J, Liebeskind JC, Able-Fessard OG (eds): *Advances in Pain Research and Therapy*. New York Raven Press, 1979, vol 3.
19. Crue BL, Felsööry A, Pinsky J: The Nashold Procedure—case report, in Crue BL (ed): *Chronic Pain*. New York, Spectrum Publications, 1979.
20. Crue BL, Todd EM: A simplified technique of sacral rhizotomy for pelvic pain. *J Neurosurg* 21:835–837, 1964.
21. Crue BL, Todd EM, Carregal EJA: Percutaneous radiofrequency stereotactic trigeminal tractotomy, in Crue BL (ed): *Pain and Suffering—Selected Aspects*. Springfield, Ill, Charles C Thomas, 1970.
22. Crue BL, Todd EM, Carregal EJA: Observations on the present status of the compression procedure in trigeminal neuralgia, in Crue BL (ed): *Pain and Suffering—Selected Aspects*. Springfield, Ill, Charles C Thomas, 1970.
23. Crue BL, Todd EM, Carregal EJA, et al: Posterior approach for high cervical percutaneous radiofrequency stereotaxic chordotomy, in Crue BL (ed): *Pain and Suffering—Selected Aspects*. Springfield, Ill, Charles C Thomas, 1970.
24. Crue BL, Todd EM, Wright WH, et al: Sacral rhizotomy for pelvic pain, in Crue BL (ed): *Pain and Suffering—Selected Aspects*. Springfield, Ill, Charles C Thomas, 1970.
25. Felsööry A, Crue BL: Results from transcutaneous high cervical electrical chordotomy, in Crue BL (ed): *Pain, Research and Treatment*. New York, Academic Press, 1975.
26. Felsööry A, Crue BL: Results of 19 years' experience with sacral rhizotomy for perianal and perineal cancer pain. *Pain* 2:431, 1976.
27. Felsööry A, Crue BL: *Neurosurgical Relief of Lumbar Spine Pain*. St. Louis, CV Mosby Co, 1981.
28. Nashold B, Crue BL: Nesencephalic and trigeminal tractotomy, in Youman's *Neurosurgery*, ed 2. Philadelphia, WB Saunders, 1981.
29. Pinsky JJ, Crue BL: Psychosurgery, in Crue BL (ed): *Chronic Pain*. New York, Spectrum Publications, 1979.
30. Wright WH, Todd EM, Crue BL, et al: Technique of transnasal stereotactic radiofrequency hypophysectomy, in Crue BL (ed): *Pain and Suffering—Selected Aspects*. Springfield, Ill, Charles C Thomas, 1970.
31. Pinsky JJ, Crue BL: Why a pain unit? in Crue BL (ed): *Chronic Pain*. New York, Spectrum Publications, 1979.
32. Pinsky JJ, Griffin, S, Agnew D, et al: Aspects of long term evaluation of pain unit treatment—CIBPS. *Bull Los Angeles Neurol Soc* 44:53, 1979.
33. Yarton P, Pinsky JJ, Crue BL: The present status of transcutaneous electrical stimulation, in Crue BL (ed): *Chronic Pain*. New York, Spectrum Publications, 1979.

34. Crue BL: Comments on recent neurochemical central brain stem aspects of pain, in Crue BL (ed): *Chronic Pain.* New York, Spectrum Publications, 1979.
35. Chauvin D: Nursing assessment of the patient with pain, in Crue BL (ed): *Pain, Research and Treatment.* New York, Academic Press, 1975.
36. Crue BL: Role of neurosurgeon on pain unit, in Crue BL (ed): *Chronic Pain.* New York, Spectrum Publications, 1979.
37. Yarton P: The role of the nurse on the pain unit, in Crue BL (ed): *Chronic Pain.* New York, Spectrum Publications, 1979.
38. Pinsky JJ: Psychodynamics and psychotherapy in the treatment of patients with chronic intractable pain. *J Human Stress* 4:17, 1978.
39. Pinsky JJ: Chronic intractable benign pain: A syndrome and its treatment with intensive short-term psychotherapy. *J Human Stress* 4:17, 1978.
40. Pinsky JJ, Crue BL, Agnew DC: *The Psychology of Chronic Pain.* New York, Spectrum Publications (submitted for publication).
41. Kübler-Ross E: *On Death and Dying.* New York, Macmillan, 1970.
42. Dolan V: A nurse looks at death and dying, in Crue BL (ed): *Chronic Pain.* New York, Spectrum Publications, 1979.
43. Worcester A: *The Care of the Aged, the Dying, and the Dead.* Springfield, Ill, Charles C Thomas, 1961.
44. Oelrich M: Working with the patient with a fatal illness, in Crue BL (ed): *Chronic Pain.* New York, Spectrum Publications, 1979.
45. Crue BL, Felsööry A, Agnew D, et al: The team concept in the management of pain in patients with cancer. *Bull Los Angeles Neurol Soc* 44:70, 1979.
46. Crue BL, Carregal EJA, Felsööry A: Percutaneous stereotaxic radiofrequency trigeminal tractotomy with neurophysiological recordings, in Crue BL (ed): *Pain, Research and Treatment.* New York, Academic Press, 1975.
47. Crue BL, Pinsky JJ, Agnew DC, et al: What is a pain center? *Bull Los Angeles Neurol Soc* 41:160, 1976.
48. Randle W: The role of the social worker as a change agent in the pain center, in Crue BL (ed): *Pain, Research and Treatment.* New York, Academic Press, 1975.
49. Randle W: Role of social service in therapy on the pain unit, in Crue BL (ed): *Chronic Pain.* New York, Spectrum Publications, 1979.
50. Felsööry A, Crue BL: Clinical results from posterior approach percutaneous stereotaxic radiofrequency high cervical chordotomy, in Crue BL (ed): *Pain, Research and Treatment.* New York, Academic Press, 1975.
51. McCaffery M: Current misconceptions about the relief of acute pain, in Crue BL (ed): *Chronic Pain.* New York, Spectrum Publications, 1979.

III

Cancer and the Health Professional

9

Cancer and the Therapy of the Word

Roger J. Bulger

Much has been made of the doctor–patient relationship over the years. Its nature, function, and desirability are under scrutiny and open to increasing questioning. Some scholars[1,2] are seeking to define more fully the essentials of a therapeutic relationship. It is the contention here that there is such a thing as a "therapeutic or healing relationship," that it is open to all participants in human interactions, and that it is especially accessible to modern physicians precisely because they are so fully armed with powerful technological interventions of potential significant benefit to the bodies of patients or sufferers who have come to them seeking repair, restoration of function, or relief from pain, discomfort, and disease. It seems to this author that these conditions are pronounced and intensified when the disease falls under the dread rubric of "cancer," especially at the present time when therapeutic advances are becoming ever more effective.

Among the several continuing threads of the history of western medicine is one concerning the place of "the word" in therapy or, put another way, of speech in the contextual relationship between patient and physician. This author predicts that the therapeutic value of the word, particularly as it relates to the speech of the physician, will be increasingly respected by clinicians in the years ahead. Further, it is this author's belief that the dynamics of the therapeutic relationship should be the subject of systematic study and analysis and that motivated, intelligent students can learn how to use speech as a therapeutic tool and avoid its adverse reactions and sometimes all-too-toxic side-effects.

Of all the clinical circumstances where the importance of the word for positive or negative impact is apparent, those that arise around the diagnosis of cancer are among the most dramatic. The very name of this fearsome set of diseases has emotional impact. Those doctors recognized by this author as being most effective at using "the word" in therapy are often people who deal frequently with patients with cancer. Doctors skilled in using talk as therapy often seem much less frustrated by the death of the patient and seem less prone to "burn-out" in the face of cancer's ravages, perhaps because they can see that their words have had beneficial effects even in the face of death and excessive suffering. It is the purpose of this chapter to highlight the history of the word as therapy and to reflect on the implication of this history on the modern conundrum of how to humanize the high-technology interventions that so characterize medicine.

Some Historical Notes

As scholars of linguistics point out, earliest human societies relied almost solely on speech to communicate. Before writing was invented, cultures were clearly oral in nature. In such civilizations for example, history was oral, with great feats being committed to memory and transmitted from one generation to the next. Even in post-Homeric ancient Greece, the great orators remained the most influential of people; the rhetorician was also the philosopher and, as exemplified by the sophists, was supposed to be the repository of all knowledge.

As writing and symbolic thinking in mathematics came to the fore, the primacy of speech was threatened and ultimately gave way to the written word. Pedro Lain Entralgo,[3] a Spanish psychiatrist and classical Greek scholar, in his book *The Therapy of the Word in Classical Antiquity,* outlines clearly the role of therapeutic speech in Greek culture, although in his view the word never fully became a therapeutic tool until Freud developed modern psychotherapy in the late nineteenth and early twentieth century.

A thousand years before Plato, Homer wrote of three different uses of the word to benefit the sick: "cheering" speech wherein the speaker encourages the diseased person and offers human support; prayers to gods beseeching their intervention on behalf of the sufferer; and magic incantations or spells which a shaman of one sort or another utilizes to cure the patient. Plato recognized the word as a therapeutic tool as described above and allowed it a place in his *Republic,* but he specifically excluded the poets and playwrights from his ideal kingdom because those writers' words excite passions in the listener, which to Plato could lead to no good end.

For Lain Entralgo, this recognition by Plato of the emotion-stirring qualities of drama and poetry established the foundation for the psychotherapeutic intervention. Aristotle explicated the value of an emotional catharsis, which people can experience by watching a play, and he believed that such releases of pent-up emotion are highly desirable and therapeutic. Lain Entralgo claims that Aristotle's treatment of poetry and the arts is sufficiently complete that the

Greeks at that point had all the intellectual substrate required to create the new field of psychotherapy. Why then, didn't it happen?

Surprisingly, the culprits seem to have been Hippocrates and his followers. Hippocrates, as we all know, emphasized careful observation and, where appropriate, specific physical intervention to cure the patient's ills. He regarded with great disfavor those who cast charms over diseases with their words; the tradition of using words to treat the sick was at cross-purposes with the budding science of medicine. The Hippocratic corpus continued this trend, in effect for centuries institutionalizing medicine as "The Silent Art," an art based on nature, observation, reasoning, and action.

Admittedly, the writings of Hippocrates and his followers are replete with explicit advice and implications regarding moral behavior, confidentiality, and even occasionally what may be considered sensitive ways to treat patients, which included decorous and appealing habits of speech. The essential thrust was clear, however, that talk cures nothing and that this great art of medicine is basically "silent."

For Lain Entralgo, it seems that all that was changed by Freud. At last, the word as a therapeutic tool was returned to the mainstream of medicine. Alas, most would agree that the reality is that such has not been the case. Psychoanalysis and psychotherapy, while shedding great light on the inner workings of the mind and providing cures and symptom amerlioration on a limited scale, cannot claim to have returned the word to an honored placed in medicine's armamentarium. First of all, Freudian psychiatrists are felt by most physicians to be outside the central core of the medical profession or at least at its fringes. Second, in mental disease as with almost all others, the fantastic advances of modern science have produced incredible new technologies for diagnosis and treatment, such that many psychiatrists have turned to chemical interventions to deal with psychic or emotional problems, thus themselves eschewing "the word" and espousing "the silent art." The majority of modern doctors, then, remain practitioners of "the silent art," essentially outside the influence of Freudian psychiatry.

On the other hand, Erik Erikson, who certainly has been influenced by Freud, has written about the healing relationship as follows:[1]

> The healer is committed to a highest good, preserving life and furthering well-being. He need not prove scientifically that these are, in fact, the highest good; rather, he is precommitted to this basic proposition while investigating what can be verified by scientific means. This, I think, is the meaning of the Hippocratic Oath. It subordinates all medical method to a humanistic ethic. [p. 73]

Erikson goes on to define the therapeutic relationship as based in trust and the principle that both doctor and patient should gain personally from the interaction. In so doing he reminds us of the phenomenon of transference, by which the patient may seek to exploit disease for regressive or infantile goals; similarly, he warns us about "counter-transference, the healer's motivation to exploit the patient's transference and to dominate or serve, possess or love him to the detriment of his true function." Erikson was addressing these comments to all doctors and was not referring only to psychiatry, so we can see that he was in effect making an attempt to extend the range of the healing interaction beyond solely medical situations.

Until this century, the western physician had relatively little in the way of effective technological intervention to offer patients. What tools the physician did have usually didn't work or were downright harmful. The idealized doctor of that age, now often envisioned as a committed humanitarian whose practice site was the patient's home, had in fact only words to offer to ameliorate suffering. The doctor offered human support; would personally stand by the patient and support and advise the family as they watched the patient through the illness.

In the 1980s, with such wonderfully effective new tools in our possession, we doctors don't need to do that sort of thing. Our first obligation is to maintain competence—an awesome responsibility these days—and that means a continuing investment in science and technology. We need to be expert in those interventions we now have at our disposal that are so effective in treating diseases or symptoms. According to our education, x-rays, hormones, chemotherapy, antidepressants, analgesics, and CAT scans are effective tools; words are not. We are, all too often, uncomfortable with words, embarrassed by or ineffectual with them, and see them as without value in the fight against a tangible disease. We are more than ever embedded in "the silent art."

All of this is disquieting somehow. Why? In part, we are disquieted because as the profession seems to be ever more effective in utilizing its science and technology, the public is increasingly critical and disaffected. We are accused of being inhumane, mechanistically oriented, and materialistic. Although most doctors realize at some level that their words can have tremendous impact, at least on some patients, it's just not a scientific thing. Most doctors have never thought, nor do they now think, of words, especially their words, as a mode of therapy.

Against this background, science is once again leading us to some new concepts that may open the way for most doctors to consider their speech therapeutically significant. Among the modern advances in neurochemistry, there are many observations relating the emotional state with the production of certain chemicals or secretion of certain hormones. For example, the endorphins of the brain establish an endogenous supply of morphine, the production of which may in fact be open to external influences such as acupuncture or shock. It thus becomes an easy thing to envision how doctors could use words as therapy, if only they knew how to affect the patient's emotional state in an appropriate manner.

There are many examples of such interventions; certainly every superior physician has experienced several. One of the purest illustrations is referred to by Norman Cousins[4] in his book *The Anatomy of an Illness,* when he quotes Bernie Lown, the noted Harvard cardiologist, on his treatment of a patient with an acute myocardial infarction. According to Dr. Lown, the most important therapeutic beginning can be for the doctor to meet his recently stricken heart patient at the Emergency Room and to tell the patient that everything is under control and that he or she will be all right. Dr. Lown seldom has to give the traditional shot of morphine to these patients, and an important initial step to recovery has been taken. In this instance, it is clear that the word and the trust relationship have been used as therapy.

Walsh McDermott, the wise clinician-scholar whose recent death has diminished our world, in what may have been his last prepared text for formal presentation,[5] analyzed what he called "samaritanism" in modern medicine, the reasons for its decline with the advent of effective technologies in medicine, and the great need for its systematic reintroduction into the average physician's bag of treatments. Dr. McDermott makes no case for "love" as the source for "samaritanism," which he refers to as those human support functions that are best carried out by the doctor. Rather, he argues that, once it is understood by the aspiring physician how important such functions can be to therapeutic success and that in addition, one cannot be a truly great physician without knowing how to facilitate and produce emotional support for the patient and family, the intelligent and ambitious student-physician will learn how to do it. McDermott argues that "samaritanism" is not an inherited trait, that altruism is not a genetically transmitted characteristic, and that its practice can be taught. In his talk entitled "Technology's Consort," there is clearly much overlap between what McDermott calls "samaritanism" and what we have been calling the therapy of the word.

Any thoughtful physician can remember instances of wishing that words spoken could be gotten back, just as one can remember wishing one could have back a drug or operation that produced an unfortunate side-effect. Again, in this author's experience, doctors frequently dealing with cancer patients are right in the thick of the issue. In the past, the diagnosis "cancer" has meant death to most patients. Now, as the disease is subdivided and various treatments are variously successful, many patients have a very good chance for survival. How and what they are told can have tremendous impact—again, both positive and negative—on patient and loved ones.

Cancer

The treatment of many cancers is now so complex that many different doctors can enter the word-therapy arena for any given patient, therein creating a potential—and sometimes very real—crisis in trust and emotional health. For example, this author has known several radiation therapists who have complained that some patients' general physicians have not adequately informed the patient and that they (the radiation therapists) are stuck at the very end of the clinical course with the unpalatable task of explaining an inevitably fatal outcome to the distraught patient. All too often, such a conversation can come out with such great statistical precision that, for all one knows, a subsequent loss of hope might in fact contribute to placing the patient among those whose therapy is not successful.

The observation that western medicine, beginning in the fifth century B.C. with Hippocrates, associated itself with action rather than words may explain what otherwise could be construed as a most peculiar and persistent separation of medicine from the great healers and healings associated with religion and religious leaders. The power of belief, whether it be in touching the prophet, going to Lourdes, or accepting Christian Science, is obviously a most powerful therapeutic tool. Although one explanation for these phenomena may be pure-and-simple divine intervention external to the patient, another may be related to the impact on the disease of an altered mental status and belief structure on the part of the patient. We tend to think of these healers and "miraculous" cures as being of the past, from the prescientific medical era, but, in fairness, even the most skeptical among us must recognize that these things continue to occur among the simple and the sophisticated, affecting people with access to all the high technology that modern medicine has to offer. Not only have we no explanation, modern science has done little to pursue possible explanations for these phenomena.

In this author's experience, there has been one extraordinary case suggesting the overbearing influence of mental factors in the course of a disease in a situation when it was quite clear that religion had little involvement. While a medical resident in the early 1960s, this author saw the x-rays of a famous patient who was being followed at the Seattle VA Hospital. The patient, a heavy smoker, went to his private physician with significant cough; an x-ray showed bilateral pulmonary infiltrates and masses, and a supraclavicular mass was palpable. The doctor told the patient that he believed he had metastatic carcinoma of the lung, that he should go down to the VA Hospital for biopsy to prove it, and that he should begin to get his affairs in order so as to prepare for an orderly transition to infinity.

The patient became incensed, grabbed his x-rays, and headed for the VA Hospital, shouting at his doctor in defiance, "I'll live to piss on your grave!" At the VA Hospital, the biopsy was positive and his lungs looked horrendous on x-ray, with one side being almost completely obliterated. The patient, an angry, uncooperative man, had one x-ray treatment session before he left the hospital against advice. On subsequent return visits for follow-up chest x-rays, his lungs cleared and ultimately there was no evidence of disease. His was a case of complete tumor regression without known treatment save the one therapeutically inconsequential x-ray treatment and possibly his Olympian anger. A year or two after his first visit to the VA Hospital, he reported that his doctor had died and he had gone out to the cemetery and urinated on his grave! I don't know whether his cancer returned after his revenge was consummated.

Anyone who has ever sacrificed experimental rats by exposure to ether in a jar knows how some fight the anesthetic far more vigorously and effectively than others. Apparently, there is some evidence that patients who get angry at having cancer fight it more effectively than do those more passive souls who seem more willing to accept death.

All these realities tend to suggest that one aim of the therapeutic relationship shall be for the physician to aid the patient in the attainment of a state of mind in which the patient may most optimally cure him- or herself or aid the external technical interventions in the curative process. To do this requires a lot more insight into and knowledge, understanding, and analysis of what makes some patients get well and others not do so and of how the doctor can influence the process through behavior and speech. There's got to be a better way than preceding the patient to the grave.

On the Word as Therapy

What is this "therapy of the word," about which we have been speaking? In this discussion, we have included Homer's "cheering speech" (which sounds like an ancient equivalent of a good bedside manner), followed Lain Entralgo's arguments about psychotherapy as word therapy, as well as all the human support functions arising from a successful doctor–patient relationship through a consideration of Walsh McDermott's idea of medical "samaritanism" and the example of Dr. Lown's approach to a patient with a myocardial infarction. Finally, we have touched upon the religious or faith-healers and implied that there may be some important linkages between them and traditional medicine.

From this author's perspective, word therapy for the physician–healer should encompass all of these dimensions. It must be emphasized that research and study must go forward in this area in order to give structure to the dialogue. In this author's current view, there are at least three different, identifiable levels of activity and positive impact upon the patient by the doctor.

The first level is the one based on an appearance of competence and a willingness to communicate with and advise the patient. There is comfort in knowing that one has a "good" doctor—one who knows what she or he is doing and yet recognizes her or his limitations and will get help as is required.

The second level comes when the doctor demonstrates she or he will stick with the patient in the most trying circumstances, attempting to get the most effective technologies brought to bear on the patient's problems and doing all that is possible to encourage the patient to do what is necessary to help him-

or herself to get better. On this level, it seems to me that Erik Erikson's concept of the golden rule becomes apparent in the healing relationship. "My doctor is working with me much as she would like to be worked with if she were in my situation," is the beneficially operative realization for the patient.

Erikson goes further in his analysis, likening the doctor–patient relationship to aspects of the parent–child interaction, which is similarly unequal. He points out that in the best parent–child relationship, both participants grow from the encounter and that trust and a mutuality of interest in a positive outcome are at the basis of a healthy interaction.

The third level would be achieved when in Erikson's words a real cure occurs; thus, "a real cure transcends the transitory state of patienthood; it is an experience which enables the cured patient to develop and to transmit to home and neighbor an attitude toward health which is one of the most essential ingredients of an ethical outlook." It is at this level that the element of faith in the physician can be most beneficial to the patient and where the realities and dangers of the processes of transference and countertransference must be appreciated fully by the doctor.

Although this level of interaction may be infrequently reached or even warranted, it is out of this kind of interaction that many truly major cures, especially those relating to major behaviorial changes on the patient's part, may be effected.

This analysis is not meant to imply that the great physician should acquire the techniques of the faith-healer or aspire to producing miracles out of the power of his or her words or personality. Rather, it is argued that the combination of the tremendous power of modern science and medical technology resting in the physician's hands and the frightening mental abyss created by a major disease for the sufferer establish the environment out of which the various levels of a healing relationship can be developed. Sensitive and motivated physicians can work at their role throughout a lifetime of practice; and, from time to time, for some patients, they can be the instrument through which a "real cure" emerges through a relationship that will be beneficial to both patient and doctor. The scientific physician-healer must remain firmly rooted in science but may be able to learn to tap some of the emotional reserves seemingly open to nontraditional healers. Therein lies a challenge that should be taken up.

In the ancient oral cultures, spoken words had an enormous power and immediacy, difficult for moderns to appreciate. The power that primitive people attached to spoken words through charms and spells, and which Hippocrates and his followers down through the present time have ascribed to magic or to religious faith, may in fact have some intelligible biochemical explanation. Today, as Professor Walter Ong says,[6]

> . . . the world moves in the new orality of our electronic era, where the telephone, loudspeaker, radio and television give voice a new kind of cur-

rency. Our new secondary orality makes us in significant ways like those who lived in the old primary oral culture. [p. 14]

One wonders, as our physical exams become more cursory and physical touching of the patient less prominent, if the verbal interchange will not become ever more important. Medicine is ready for a new look at the use of the word in treatment. The subject needs exploration and analysis; it needs to be expanded conceptually beyond classical psychotherapy; it needs emphasis and it needs to be taught wherever it can be. There is no more apt place for this to go on than at the clinical interface between the patient and doctor dealing with cancer.

References

1. Erikson EH: The golden rule and the cycle of life, in Bulger RJ (ed): *Hippocrates Revisited.* New York, Medcom Press, 1973.
2. Pellegrino ED, Thomasma, DC: *A Philosophical Basis of Medical Practice.* New York and Oxford, Oxford University Press, 1981.
3. Entralgo, PL: *The Therapy of the Word in Classical Antiquity.* New Haven and London, Yale University Press, 1970.
4. Cousins, N: *The Anatomy of an Illness as Perceived by the Patient.* New York, W.W. Norton and Co., 1979, p 135–136.
5. McDermott W, Rogers D: Technology's Consort, paper presented at the Johnson Foundation Clinical Scholar Annual Meeting, San Antonio, October 1981.
6. Ong W: In Entralgo PL: *The Therapy of the Word in Classical Antiquity.* New Haven and London, Yale University Press, 1970.

10

The Doctor–Patient Relationship in Oncology: Implications for Practice, Research, and Policy Planning

Arthur S. Levine

Recent changes in the quality of our society and culture have profoundly affected health care. From my vantage point at the National Institutes of Health, it is possible to view these changes with considerable clarity, for the NIH reflects the quintessence of such new issues as high technology and its cost; informed consent; the rapidity with which the results of basic research should be applied at the bedside; the increasing influence of regulatory law, economics, and politics on health care; and today's culture of consumerism and its influence on research priorities.

Another, and I believe the most important issue with which I have dealt as a physician in the National Cancer Institute, is that of the doctor-patient relationship. Here, too, great change has occurred, and the expectancy for cure, now often implicit in a patient's referral to the NCI or other prominent cancer center, permits one to bring into sharp focus the characteristics that have defined this relationship in the past and now appear to be redefining it. To a large extent, the physician-patient relationship must be at the heart of our concern with evolution in medical practice, research, and policy planning. It is proposed here that the more commonly discussed issues of the cost:benefit ratio of high technology, the establishment of research priorities, and informed consent are only variations on the theme of this relationship.

Historically, the most severe problem for physicians has been the formation of dependency relationships with their patients.[1] In the NCI clinical oncology fellowship training program, we have taken up this issue both practically and theoretically, using classic studies of group behavior as guides. In this rubric, the physician may be substituted for "leader," with patients comprising "the group." Members of any group have the tendency to divest themselves of large portions of their individual autonomy by projecting it upon the designated leader. In this way, the leader is considered responsible for the group's fate and, therefore, must take care of it in every imaginable way.[2] Historically, this dynamic endowed the physician (who believed it!) with glamour, nobility, exceptional authority, and indeed supernatural powers. In the early part of this century, the authority of science was added to that of the doctor's white coat to validate this image. The physician became an active scientist, while the patient remained passive material.

More recently, however, it has followed from these dependency relationships that if the giver of care is found derelict in any capacity, this individual's utility as a leader is at an end. In this more-than-lifesize role, it is almost impossible to avoid a misstep. When the misstep occurs, not only may the physician's utility be found wanting, but it actually may be perceived that he should be destroyed. There is no more extreme instance of guilt than that commonly displayed by the family of a patient whose life is threatened. One method for diminishing the anxiety produced by this guilt is the use of a "scapegoat." All the power of the intellect and profound attention to detail is brought to bear on the selection of the scapegoat, since, to be effective in reducing anxiety, the scapegoat must be part of a rational, credible system. Like religious converts, patient and family must convince nurses, doctors, other patients—and ultimately lawyers—of their belief in the dereliction of the chosen doctor. In its extreme form, this process can have a devastating effect on the patient and the physician alike.

Why have doctors entered relationships that promote scapegoating? One may extrapolate from our model of group and leader to the situation in which a patient or family attempts to pursuade the physician to enter a subtle, often unvoiced, contract, with the good or flattering patient rewarded with a cure. The patient says, "Between you and me and God, we'll make it, won't we, Doc?" In an instant, the physician accepts this contract. When the relationship has expanded and become a reality between the two, doctors find themselves in a wholly anomalous situation—they are made to feel that they have in fact promised a cure. When they are not able to produce one, it follows that they have been negligent in their duties. Physicians are puzzled and disturbed by the extent of their own guilt feelings, wherein they accuse themselves of failing. When the process is complete, the patient has pursuaded the doctor that if death or complications occur, they will be due to "inadequate doctoring," rather than to illness. Thus, the physician (and often the nurse) is perfectly set up for severe depression, if indeed the patient does die or if severe complications develop.

Nearly every physician and many nurses have a large element of the hero in their self-concepts. In fact, this quality is vital to getting them into and through the rigors of medical or nursing training. The notion of heroism is a particular liability because this quality makes the physician particularly susceptible to the patient's praise and flattery. It is easy for physicians to come to expect a "larger-than-life" performance from themselves. Sadly, the results of dependency relationships between professionals and patients, and the subtle contracts for complication-free cures that doctors permit as a function of their heroism, serve to compromise the patient in the end, for the role of hero is basically untenable. It produces anxiety and guilt. To avoid these uncomfortable feelings, doctors often isolate patients and their families, denying them the humanism that is their due, and the doctors' as well.

The heroic posture also precludes doctors from dealing effectively with the role of society as a concomitant to illness, because doctors cannot be sensitive to the currents of society if they float in an ark while everyone else is swimming. As Erik Erikson has noted, the psyche, the soma, and society all impact on one another.[1] The fact frequently has been overlooked that families and even whole neighborhoods must undertake a series of rituals when one member becomes seriously ill or is threatened with death. For example, many physicians are unaware of the possibility of profound community reaction to the diagnosis of cancer. That very word is a cultural metaphor, replacing the nineteenth century's use of the word "consumption," as described by Susan Sontag,[3] yet physicians profess surprise when offered the observation that cancer frequently is still seen as a disgrace or a punishment for misdeeds. Not being aware of these social phenomena, physicians often have serious altercations with members of the patient's family as misunderstandings accumulate. The staff resorts to repeating medical facts while the family pleads with them for social solutions to their community problems.

These social phenomena are particularly evident in my own clinical setting, that of childhood cancer.[4] Parents almost always feel a fair burden of guilt when childhood cancer is diagnosed. They believe that everyone is watching and taking note of their neglect, and often there is information to fuel the fire: The ill child may have been the product of an unwanted pregnancy, there may have been a divorce, the parents may have been preoccupied with their careers, or the child may not have received timely immunizations. There are countless pieces of information that will serve the purposes of this all-consuming guilt. However, the family almost invariably does not express these uncomfortable feelings in terms of their content as such but rather in the form of medical jargon that they feel is the only permissible means of communication between themselves and their physicians. Time after time, doctors specifically misunderstand the parents' request for information about their seriously ill child, responding with medical data when the parents really want to discuss their own sense of guilt and complicity in the cancer. Although physicians do recognize that they are being asked to listen and to enter into a human equation with their patients and their patients' families, there is an almost universal fear of entering such discussions. The staff will usually say, "If I once let it get started, I'll never get anything else done." We fear being overwhelmed, and in trying to avoid personal and intimate issues, we frequently consume more time than we would use in simply listening.

So far, our concern here has been with dependency relationships between physicians and patients, brought on by historical perceptions of the doctor as hero and the psychological needs of patients and their families in times of suffering and stress. Almost as an attempted antidote to these historical relationships, and to the increasing dehumanization of modern medical practice, change has arrived in the name of *holism,* a new humanistic attempt to keep body and soul together, not only now, but forever. As Christopher Lasch tells us,[5] there is a connection between "the clinical aspects of the narcissistic syndrome" and "certain characteristic patterns of contemporary culture," such as our intense fear of old age and death. In our time, God, the flag, the military, our political leadership, and the medical establishment have excited the loyalty and enthusiasm of fewer and fewer citizens. What is left for them but themselves? An endless series of fads seems to have as its object self-promotion and self-enhancement. Not the least of these fads is our willingness as a society to spend $100 billion on health care, despite the fact that much of this cost represents an effort to compensate for the incapacitating effects of certain diseases whose course we are largely unable to alter.[6] Certain aspects of the interferon "growth-industry," chemical carcinogenesis research, diet and nutrition studies, and federally funded clinical trials of agents for which there is no preclinical promise, all reflect this situation. The paradox of clinical research "fads" is that true insight into disease comes slowly, unpredictably, often ungovernably, and often at random. Moreover, the fruits of basic research cannot be legislated, nor can they be bribed, above a certain threshold level of funding. But when the fruits come, the cost of so-called high technology disappears as, for instance, with the cost of polio vaccine versus that of iron lungs.

This new, narcissistic view of health care also emphasizes, in an age of consumerism, the individual patient's responsibility as an initiating participant in her or his own health care. In contrast to society's earlier view of the physician as omnipotent, we now question the doctor's every move, as well as those of the medical profession in its entirety and the biomedical research establishment. Often, hospitals are accused of prolonging agony, rather than renewing life. Furthermore, we have begun to exhort patients to become active warriors in the good fight against their diseases.[7] The new trend seems to me, in part, to be a good one. For far too long, people have been excluded from the care and maintenance of their own minds and bodies, equally victimized by prescriptions written in Latin and by manipulative television commercials. Unfortunately, one cannot suddenly awake and assume self-responsibility; instead, it takes training from earliest childhood, with virtually a lifetime of experience, independence, and maturation. The skills of responsibility are complex; one must be able to analyze the variable forces around oneself and to exercise great competence in assessing options so as to modify one's personal strengths and weaknesses.

When society begins to extol self-reliance to people who, throughout their lives, have been so manipulated that they now lack the skills of self-reliance, the result is self-accusation, not self-responsibility.[8] Patients and families in this situation will ascribe the illness to a failure of willpower: "Somehow, we did this to ourselves; it's all our fault." These kinds of feelings clearly undermine the possibility of good medical care. To the degree that we, as professionals, join the general exhortation, we encourage in our patients and their families a sense of abandonment and worthlessness. Surely, there can be nothing more isolating than to imply to patients and families that they are now responsible for the outcome of the illness, when they lack the lifetime of competence necessary to assume any part of this responsibility. But our spurious preoccupation with self-reliance grows. We are told to battle our cancer cells, and "will" our white blood cell count into rising! We charge ahead, determined to conquer nature in all of its forms, including illness, aging, and death. Such a preoccupation seems to me to be particularly American. Since we long have had the resources with which to accomplish so much, surely there is no stopping us now! We would do well to listen to other cultures, which may have a superior philosophy. They agree that we should not yield to illness, nor should we accept death with grace. But when we uncritically join the cry for inappropriate self-reliance, we demonstrate our inability to recognize the limits of people's power over themselves, limits that are inherent in the human condition.

There is, of course, an ultimate paradox in our all-consuming desire to be in control of our lives, our deaths, and our universe. No matter how much we jog, clean the rivers, purify the air, drink Perrier, hold our doctors accountable, and weigh carefully the options offered by "informed consent," our mortality rate will still be 100 percent. We cannot seriously postpone the inevitable process of aging and decay, despite the fact that our society surrounds us with manufactured fantasies of total and perennial gratification and the myth that we only die because we get sick. Meanwhile, as Lewis Thomas has written so eloquently, we are paying too little attention and respect to the built-in durability and sheer power of the human organism and its surest tendency toward stability and balance. It is a distortion, with something profoundly disloyal about it, to picture the human being as a teetering, fallible contraption, always needing watching, patching, and a nearby Health Maintenance Organization. Instead, we should celebrate the marvel of good health that is really the lot of most of us, most of the time.[6]

Thus, the recent change in our society's view of the patient as a powerful, self-reliant, but suspicious consumer, brings us full circle to the notion of omnipotence in medical care. Only now, it is the patient (or his family) who is omnipotent and not the doctor. We must not decry this trend altogether. Patients have a right to know why they are sick and why they may die. They need to learn to take responsibility for influencing all of these aspects of their lives and deaths, and they need to engage their doctors and nurses in meaningful discussions. However, we must remember the limits of responsibility, and our mutual responsibility as related human beings. If this recent change from omnipotent physician to omnipotent patient forces professionals into greater accountability as humanists, it will be to the good, for in the past professionals often have found themselves uneasy when close to their patients, all too often avoiding the patient and finding excuses to be busy with something else when the patient expected to see them. This feeling of discomfort is particularly acute when a young physician has to deal with an adolescent or another young adult. These feelings are even more painful when there are other points of identity such as social origin and educational level. In my own setting of pediatric oncology, I have found that the physician's discomfort tends to be especially acute when the physician has a child of similar age.[4]

How can one explain the observation that physicians too often back away from their patients? It seems to me that the explanation lies within the rubric of identification. Physicians must first permit sufficient proximity with their patients to develop a sense of identity with them. However, having made this identification, they become fearful and anxious and once again wish to separate themselves from their patients. The experience of threatened death among their patients weakens physicians' defensive armor against the issue of death in their own lives, and so they are thrown into conflict. On one hand, they long for the peace of mind that they possessed before they began to confront death, but, on the other hand, they are driven by their own curiosity and sense of heroism to explore this conventionally unknown territory. As Ernest Becker has written. "Man is literally split in two: he has an awareness of his own splendid uniqueness in that he sticks out of nature with a towering majesty, and yet he goes back into the ground a few feet in order blindly and dumbly to rot and disappear forever. It is a terrifying dilemma to be in and to have to live with . . . to live a whole lifetime with the fate of death haunting one's dreams and even the most sun-filled days."[9:89]

The physician's attempt to confront the gap between human needs and an unreasonably unresponsive world commonly is represented by the question, "What should I say to the patient who may die? What can I say to give the patient and his family hope?" In fact, often there is nothing to say. As death approaches, a patient may come to accept its imminence psychologically. One consequence of this acceptance is a dramatic change in the patient's pattern of communication. For example, having no future, the patient is not interested in discussing anything that bears implications for the future—such as what the weather will be next week, or how the Redskins will do next season—leaving this person with virtually nothing to talk about. Unprepared for this phenomenon and heavily oriented by his training to provide patients with hopeful words about the future, the physician may experience a sense of helpless, almost foolish, embarrassment. Doctors' concern with the question of how to give hope, or the possibility that they may be taking away hope, seems to me to be a reflection of their own narcissism, their perception that they are so omnipotent that it is within the power of their words to alter the course of people's lives or their perception of their lives. Usually, doctors require encouragement to notice that their presence, even without any words, may be as helpful to their patients as were talking and listening earlier on.

Seeing existences terminate about them, doctors usually become quite reflective about their own. As their work proceeds, their older patients' discussions of how fully they have lived their lives have a profound effect upon them and direct them toward their own question, "Am I fulfilling my potential?" In fact, the anxiety inherent in this question is a liberating one for the doctors charged with the care of a seriously ill or dying patient, since it forces them to enter the human equation with their patients as they confront the basic issues of their own lives.

"Man does not really begin to live until he has begun to take his own mortality seriously."[10:308] This is as true for the doctor as it is for the patient. When our society finally accepts this thought and integrates it into its culture, the best of all possible changes will be at hand, from omnipotent doctor to omnipotent patient to a relationship in which neither is omnipotent, instead both are in it together. Such a change frequently will require painstaking and explicit discussion and negotiation as to the exact roles the patient, physician, and family will take. But, when we are truly partners—doctor and patient, doctor and family, doctor and nurse—then we shall have changed from the hierarchy of Martin Buber's "I-It" to the "I-Thou" relation he offered us with such elegance and purpose.[11]

The implications of the statements put forth here seem evident with respect to patient care, but perhaps less direct with regard to research priorities and policy planning. Again, it seems that the same issues of dependency, heroism, and inappropriate self-reliance are everywhere at play: They create unrealistic expectations and distrust in the public and a consequent regulatory bureaucracy that may produce stagnation in clinical research and costly defensiveness in physicians. What are the possible solutions? I believe that the way should be led by the physician in his classic role of docent or teacher. Further, one might begin with a consideration of the personalities of those who are admitted into medical schools in the first place: Excellence in the rote sciences does not predict maturity and humanism; we must enlarge our notion of who may become a good doctor and realign our medical school admissions policies. Moreover, once enrolled, the formal training of a medical student from her freshman year onward also should be concerned with the social, psychological, political, and philosophic dynamics of the doctor-patient relationship, as contrasted with the limited medical model for psychiatric illness as existing "in the patient" per se. Student-patient interactions should be supervised and analyzed by physicians who are formally trained in this approach. These mentors should represent a diversity of the primary clinical specialties and not be limited to liaison psychiatrists, such that role modeling has its fullest chance to flourish. The interpersonal skills, sensitivity, and caring necessary for rapport between doctor and patient should be emphasized in continuing medical education programs throughout the physician's career.[12] Seminars on the doctor–patient relationship, such as we have had for a number of years at the National Cancer Institute,[1] can be undertaken at each new developmental stage of a physician's working lifetime.

Finally, just as patients and physicians alike must discuss and negotiate their roles fully and honestly, so must this discussion extend to those who set policy and priority in health care and research. The bureaucracy of informed consent, with its inherent limitations of bias, misinformation, and paternalism,[13] and the laundered formalism of courses on thanatology, will not substitute for this painstaking and explicit discussion of the doctor–patient relationship and how the myths and fantasies of that relationship, and its asymmetries of power and risk, may influence so expensively and destructively every aspect of medicine and medical research. Open and mutual dialogue with the public is a *sine qua non*; just as the doctor must be a docent, the patient also must "prescribe for the physician." Moreover, just as idiosyncratic features of personality and experience may preclude the practicing physician from effectively acting upon his understanding of the doctor-patient relationship, to the point where psychotherapy for that physician becomes a strong consideration, so it may be that crises in cancer care policy and research priorities, when they occur, should be explicated with the principle of preventive and social psychiatry.

References

1. Artiss KL, Levine AS: Doctor–patient relation in severe illness. A seminar for oncology fellows. *New Engl J of Med* 288:1210–1214, 1973.
2. Bion WR: *Experiences in Groups and Others Papers.* New York, Basic Books, 1961, pp 105–113.
3. Sontag S: *Illness and Metaphor.* New York, Farrar Straus and Giroux, 1978, pp 5–9.
4. Levine AS, Artiss KL, Susman EJ: The impact of childhood cancer on doctors and nurses, in *Proceedings of the American Cancer Society National Conference on the Care of the Child with Cancer.* Philadelphia, George F. Stickley Co, 1979, pp 137–143.
5. Lasch C: *The Culture of Narcissism: American Life in an Age of Diminishing Expectations.* New York, Norton, 1979, pp 125–140.
6. Thomas L: *The Lives of a Cell.* New York, Viking Press, 1974, pp 81–86.
7. Fiore N: Fighting cancer—one patient's perspective. *New Engl J of Med* 301:284–289, 1979.
8. Shapiro DH Jr: The psychology of responsibility. *New Engl J of Med* 301: 211–212, 1979.

9. Becker E: *The Denial of Death.* New York, The Free Press–Macmillan, 1973.
10. Kaufmann WA (ed): *Existentialism from Dostoevsky to Sartre.* Cleveland, World Publishing Company, 1956, pp 221, 307–311.
11. Buber M: *I and Thou.* New York, Scribner's, 1970.
12. Jensen PS: The doctor-patient relationship: Headed for impasse or improvement? *Ann Intern Med* 95:769–771, 1981.
13. Cross AW, Churchill LR: Ethical and cultural dimensions of informed consent. A case study and analysis. *Ann Intern Med* 96:110–113, 1982.

11

The Hospice Movement and Its Relationship to Active Treatment

Irwin H. Krakoff

The development of hospice care, pioneered in England by Saunders and adopted enthusiastically in the United States and elsewhere, is providing attention and some solutions to a problem that has been seriously neglected in the past. As Saunders[1] has pointed out, straightforward acknowledgment of the fact of dying has encouraged realistic approaches to the psychological and physical needs of patients with advanced disease.

Heinemann,[2] commenting on the development of the modern hospital, has pointed out that it is economically unsound to use, for the custodial care of incurable, terminally ill patients, the expensive, elaborate facilities designed for diagnosis and active treatment. He also has noted the frustrations of the medical staff in that setting and their consequent rejection of the dying.

It appears clear that the hospital currently is not geared to the provision of optimal care for patients for whom no active therapy is planned, whether those patients have advanced cancer, neurologic disease, or some other affliction.

Much has been made of inappropriate overtreatment, and medicine has been castigated as technologically oriented, unfeeling, and concerned with preserving life to the exclusion of concern for the quality of life. The hospice thus has been promoted as an alternative care system. It is clear that Saunders always has advocated a continuing interface of the hospice with acute care. Her representation of the relationship between the "cure system" and the "care system" indicates that the heavier traffic is toward the "care system."[1] Nevertheless, there is provision for a return trip. Similarly, she has indicated an area of overlap in decisions between the two systems.

Unfortunately there seems to exist a very vocal school that does not advocate integration of Dr. Saunders' two systems but apparently wants to alienate the hospice movement from the mainstream of medical care.

In the last several years, we have seen the development of a "death and dying" cult that is antitherapy and antitherapist. Its members profess to believe that the medical profession should be excluded from management of the "terminally ill." These "patient advocates" often fail to recognize that oncologists who are technically skilled also have genuine humanitarian concern for their patients. One hears that active therapy for patients with advanced disease may deprive them of "death with dignity." Lay publications graphically portray the plight of the terminal patient with tubes in every orifice and decry the dehumanization of medicine. Not only lay people but physicians, nurses, and others in the medical profession may become very antagonistic toward the use of active therapy. Such antagonism may be inappropriate, since withholding therapy frequently can be a serious mistake. A prominent hospice proponent has recently published this statement: "There comes a time for everyone when the machines need to be turned off, the tubes removed, the medical staff chased out of the room and, if they choose, when the dying person, family and friends can be together."

Is there really a time when the medical staff should be "chased out of the room?" That is a very doubtful proposition. Admittedly, some have been insufficiently attentive to all of the needs of patients with advanced, mortal disease, and some have been guilty of therapeutic excesses. To the extent that those errors exist, they should be corrected. However, it appears that some of those who have embraced the hospice concept ardently are using it as a vehicle for their antiestablishment feelings. In their excesses they may harm the hospice movement and some of the dying.

In this author's estimation, there is in all real hospice systems acknowledgement of and provision for an interface with acute care. Dr. Saunders has noted[1] that "effective control of symptoms may accompany or revive the prospect of further treatment." The outlook for patients with progressive cancer is not necessarily entirely hopeless. There may be important diagnostic, therapeutic, and palliative measures that can be taken. Our efforts should be aimed not only at easing patients out of the world but also, when appropriate, at restoring them to an active role in it. In seeking "death with dignity" we may overlook treatable disease and provide patients with the indignity of premature death.

In a previous paper[3] this author quoted several anecdotes concerning patients, all obvious candidates for terminal care, who with further active investigation, were shown not to have cancer at all or to have cancer which, when actively treated, was compatible with several years of active, productive, comfortable life. It is not necessary to review those anecdotes here. In that paper, the concern was for the identification of the terminally ill and the neglect of those who might not be quite ready to die. This author continues to be concerned about the hazards of isolation of patients with advanced cancer or other chronic disease from the mainstream of medicine.

We also must be concerned about the alienation of such patients from participation in trials of new therapies. The identification of a patient as refractory to current conventional therapy cannot be equated automatically with referral to a terminal care facility; while some patients will choose the romanticized, graceful death at home surrounded by loving family, many opt to receive a new drug, then under study, even when well informed of its potential side-effects and the very slight possibility of benefit. Administration of experimental drugs to such patients is not exploitation; it is an entirely appropriate move, beneficial to society and to the patient. Such patients are receiving the absolute best of medical care, attention to all facets of their illnesses, and the distinct possibility of benefit from the agent under study.

A few years ago a disturbing paper appeared in the New England Journal of Medicine,[4] the first sentence of which was, "Physicians have been accused of prolonging life at any cost." The paper reported the results of a study of "extended-care facilities" in Seattle. One hundred and ninety patients who developed fever were reviewed: 109 were treated actively with antibiotics, hospitalization, or both; 9 percent of those died. Eighty-one were not given active treatment, and 59 percent of those died. The authors analyzed the status of those who did and did not receive active treatment, and the data clearly showed that "the more nursing care the patient required, the more likely he or she was not to be treated." They also noted that "nurses working in extended-care facilities usually shoulder much of the responsibility for making decisions. . . ."

That is, of course, not hospice care, but it is a kind of "care" for people with advanced disease; it is isolated from the mainstream of medicine, and the factors that went into the decision-making process somehow produced a difference of 50 percent in mortality. What are those factors? We don't really know, but the uncomfortable feeling is that they may relate less to the burden of life on a patient than to the burden of care on the attending staff. This interpretation may be incorrect, but it seems clear that, if we do have compassion for patients with advanced disease, decisions regarding their care must be made in the mainstream, not apart from it, and the propriety of technical support and of restoration to active function must remain an option.

Patients with advanced cancer may exhibit many problems resulting directly from the cancer. These include pain; anemia; infection; weight loss; effusion into pleural, peritoneal, or pericardical spaces; and uremia, hypercalcemia, and other metabolic abnormalities. Any one of these could be viewed as a prospective terminal event. However, it is important both to differentiate and to understand what is truly terminal and what is reversible. We often can restore patients to reasonable health even in the presence of metastatic cancer.

It also is important to remember that cancer does not confer immunity to other disease, which may be treatable and, if properly diagnosed and treated, reversible. We can treat cardiovascular disease, infections, and so on, but this requires a frame of mind in which one asks, "What is causing this problem and what can be done about it?" rather than accepts physical deterioration as an expected, even welcome, phenomenon.

Approximately half of the patients with advanced cancer have pain as a prominent feature of their disease. It has been emphasized repeatedly that regular, anticipatory administration of analgesic drugs provides better relief from pain than if drugs are given after pain recurs. In much of the hospice promotions, it has been stated that only in the hospice setting can appropriate scheduling of pain medications be accomplished. It should be clear that there is no inconsistency between active treatment and good pain control and that pain control is achieved by intelligent management of that problem regardless of where it is done.

At the Vermont Regional Cancer Center we have had a program[5] for the last four years in which we have studied the role of nurses, social workers, nutritionists, physical therapists, and clergy in the management of patients with advanced cancer in the home as an integral part of an active, broad-based oncology service. Those patients have moved freely between home, outpatient clinic, and hospital, as required by medical and psychosocial factors. About one-third of the patients died at home, and many of the others spent only the last two or three days in the hospital. Those patients and their families benefited from the compassion of the support team and never sacrificed the technical resources of the major medical center. The dollar cost of the program is far less than hospital, nursing home, or institutional hospice programs; the benefits in patient and family well-being appear no less impressive.

In the development of drugs or other new methods of treatment, we long ago adopted a scientific approach to the evaluation of the new methods. We have set up systems of evaluating, recording, and communicating the toxicity of a new drug and the degree and regularity with which it produces regression of tumor masses or prolongation of survival.[6,7] We have developed systems of notations[8] that describe the functional ability of patients, and we have examined those systems for accuracy and reproducibility.[9] The hope that a new drug will be beneficial is meaningless, whether that drug be nitrogen mustard or Laetrile. What is significant is the objective demonstration that it is beneficial. Similarly, although the good intentions of the hospice movement are evident, one may hesitate at the automatic assumption that the results are good. Just as the clinical investigator must prove the merit of his new treatment, the hospice people must now prove the merit of their new treatment. The fact that such measurements are difficult makes them no less necessary. If our society is to move into wholesale employment of hospices, we should do so on the basis that the hospice can be proven to deal with the problems in its defined areas of interest more effectively than other medical facilities and that it does not deprive patients of necessary, appropriate medical care.

One of the straw men that some of the isolationists have set up is the concept that in the medical establishment there are two mutually exclusive goals: (1) cure or (2) abandonment. That concept is incorrect. It is incumbent on us to eradicate disease when we can; however, we recognize that there are many instances in which that is not possible. The entire field of medical oncology has been developed to deal with the problems of patients with advanced cancer. We can cure a few, we can prolong survival in some, and we can improve the quality of survival in many. Radiation oncology, an older discipline, has a similar orientation, and cancer surgery often has appropriately palliative aims. We do recognize that there are patients whose death is imminent, but, even for those, substantial comfort can be provided with the technology that is rejected by the isolationists. The pain of a bony metastasis that requires large doses of narcotics (Brompton's cocktail or others) often can be relieved by simple, low-dose radiotherapy. Dehydration is unpleasant; thus, the administration of 1500 ml of fluids intravenously daily can be a compassionate, humanitarian maneuver, not a fiendish exhibition of technical virtuosity. Intestinal obstruction with vomiting and abdominal distension is not conducive to a good quality of life; thus, the intern with a nasogastric tube is not attacking a patient, he is providing comfort and relief. After decompression with that tube (a simple maneuver) a patient can relax and enjoy the presence of his family, and vice versa.

If a multidisciplinary team approach is to be used (and there is no doubt that patient care should be multidisciplinary), the team must include the physician, who must use all of the tools at her or his disposal to accomplish the legitimate aims of treatment. Further, although patients with cancer are not the only potential clients of the hospice system, they do constitute a major segment, and for those patients care must be provided or coordinated by those with a good background in cancer medicine.

The development of oncologic specialties in medicine is part of the same recognition of needs of patients with advanced cancer as is the growth of the hospice movement. Technologic capability is neither bad nor unfeeling. Technical skill and compassion need not and should not be separate. Isolation of patients with advanced disease will deprive them of appropriate technology. Further, as social agencies and insurors recognize the need and obligation to provide services for patients with advanced disease, there will be competition between systems for the health care dollars if there are separate systems. That may be good for some of the health industry entrepreneurs but it can only be bad for our patients.

References

1. Saunders CM: Appropriate Treatment, Appropriate Death in the Management of Terminal Disease, CM Saunders, (ed), London, Edward Arnold Ltd, 1978.

2. Heinemann HO: Incurable illness and the hospital in the twentieth century. *Man and Medicine* 1:281–285, 1976.

3. Krakoff IH: The case for active treatment in patients with advanced cancer: Not everyone needs a hospice. *Ca* 29:108–111, 1979.

4. Brown NK, Thompson DJ: Nontreatment of fever in extended-care facilities. *New England J. Med.* 300:1246–1250, 1979.

5. Yates JW, Kun L, McKegney PF: Team care of patients with advanced cancer: A comparative study. Submitted for publication, 1980.

6. Krakoff IH: Clinical techniques for evaluating antineoplastic drugs in animal and clinical pharmacologic techniques, in Nodine JH, Siegler PE (eds): *Drug Evaluation.* Year Book Medical Publishers, 1964, pp 632–639.

7. Carter SK, Babowski MT, Hellman K: *Chemotherapy of Cancer.* New York, John Wiley, 1977.

8. Karnofsky DA, Burchenal JH: The clinical evaluation of chemotherapeutic agents in cancer, in MacLeod CM (ed): *Evaluation of Chemotherapeutic Agents.* New York, Columbia University Press, 1949, pp 191–205.

9. Yates JW, Chalmer B, McKegney PF: Evaluation of patients with advanced cancer using the Karnofsky Performance Status. *Cancer* 45:228–232, 1980.

IV

Cancer and
the Individual

12

Confrontation with Cancer: Historical and Existential Aspects

Carl G. Kardinal and Bruce N. Strnad

> I am troubled; I am bowed down greatly; I go mourning all the day long. For my loins are filled with a loathsome disease and there is no soundness in my flesh. [Psalm 38:6,7]

The confrontation with a life-threatening disease such as cancer precipitates a myriad of simultaneous reactions in the host. These reactions and the individual's ability to cope with them to a large degree are defined historically, culturally, educationally, and theologically. This is not to say that individuals do not react uniquely, but they react uniquely within a culturally dependent context. Human suffering and pain have biological, physical, pathological, psychological, and sociological aspects; therefore, the understanding of an individual's reaction to a confrontation with cancer must include much more than a knowledge of molecular biology, pharmacology, and radiation physics. Understanding must include the meaning of cancer to the individual and the meaning of cancer within his historical and cultural context.

Although public attitudes are changing gradually, there still are feelings that cancer is totally incurable, horribly painful, and always fatal. Cancer is the disease that "doesn't knock before it enters."[1] A sense of shame and contamination are associated with cancer. This is perpetuated too often by the well-meaning physician who will state, for example, that the chest x-ray was "clean," implying that if cancer were present it would have been "dirty." Cancer is a disease that no one has managed to glamorize. No one conceives of cancer as a "decorous" or "lyrical" way to die, because cancer patients "shrivel" and "shrink" away.[1]

In order to treat the cancer patient effectively, one must attempt to understand the crisis, the terror, the helplessness, the despair, and the perceived curse of the disease. One must attempt to ameliorate suffering through understanding.

Historical Aspects

Humankind has been aware of the existence of cancer since the beginning of recorded history. Tumors were described in the ancient Egyptian papyri dating back to 1600 B.C. The following is an excerpt from the Edwin Smith Papyrus translated by Henry Breasted.[2]

Title

Instructions concerning bulging tumors on his breast.

Examination

If thou examinest a man having bulging tumors on his breast, [and] thou findest that [swellings] have spread over his breast; if thou puttest thy hand upon his breast upon these tumors, [and] thou findest them very cool, there being no fever at all therein when thy hand touches him, they have no granulation, they form no fluid, they do not generate secretions of fluid, and they are bulging to thy hand,

Diagnosis

Thou shouldst say concerning him: One having bulging tumors. An ailment which I will contend.

Treatment

There is no [treatment].

This excerpt is confirmation that the ancient Egyptians were not only aware of breast cancer, but considered it incurable.

People always have required explanations for things they could not understand. Of necessity, these explanations have been restricted to the philosophic, theologic, and scientific knowledge of the day and have been forced into that conceptual framework.[3] This overwhelming need to find an explanation is a response to the discomfort we feel when confronted with an unknown. The correctness of the explanation does not necessarily affect the sense of satisfaction the answer gives,[4] as the following examples demonstrate.

Humoral Theory of Cancer

Over the centuries, various concepts of cancer were proposed as a means of explaining the disease to the physicians and patients of the period. The first major concept of cancer originated in ancient Greece. Greek medicine was strongly influenced by Platonic and Aristotelian thought and was expressed within that context. According to Hippocrates (c. 400 B.C.) the body was composed of four basic humors: blood, phlegm, yellow bile, and black bile. Excesses or deficiencies, or sequestrations of one or more of these were the causes of disease. Cancer was thought to be caused by an excess of black bile (atrabilis).[3,5]

Since cancer was caused by the excess of a basic body humor, it was by definition a systemic disease affecting the entire body, a systemic disease that could not be cured by local forms of treatment. The popular belief that surgery may make cancers worse dates back over 2000 years to Hippocrates, who stated that deep-seated tumors should never be operated upon as the operation might make them worse and the patient might indeed die more quickly.

Hippocrates was the first to use the term carcinoma (karkinoma), derived from karkinos (crab). The analogy of the disease to the crab was thus established:

Cancer is a rounded, unequal, hard, livid tumor, generally seated in the glandulus parts of the body, supposed to be so called because it appears at length with turgid veins shooting out from it, so as to resemble the figure of a crab; or as others say, because like a crab, where it has once got, it is scarce possible to drive it away.[6:59]

Galen (c. 200 A.D.) expanded the humoral theory and further emphasized the systemic nature of cancer. Galen classified tumors into three groups as follows:

1. *Supra naturum* (exceeding nature), such as the callus formation uniting a fracture
2. *Secundam naturum* (according to nature), such as the gravid uterus, or the swelling of breast tissue during puberty
3. *Praeter naturum* (contrary to nature), including true tumors, edema, phlegmon and gangrene.[7]

Cancer Initially a Local Disease

Galenic theory dominated medicine for the next 1300 years, establishing Galen as the most influential physician of all time. Throughout the entire Middle Ages, Galen was not to be questioned. It was only after the meticulous anatomic studies of Andreas Vesalius (c. 1540) failed to confirm the existence of black bile, that the humoral theory of cancer could be challenged effectively.

During the next 150 years, there was a gradual conceptual change from cancer as a systemic humoral disease to cancer as an initially localized disease. The strongest individual force in this change was Henri Francois LeDran (1685–1770). After performing many autopsies and anatomical studies, he was convinced that breast cancer was a localized disease in its early stages and spread via lymphatics to regional lymph nodes. But if a drop of "cancer lymph" passed the adjacent nodes it contaminated the entire system.[3,5]

The concept that cancer is initially a localized disease has enormous psychosocial implications.[8] If cancer starts locally and later invades, there is some chance for cure with local treatment. With LeDran's observations, it was possible to counter the absolute hopelessness inherent in the humoral theory. Hope for therapy replaced the belief that cancer was incurable.

The first edition of the *Encyclopaedia Britannica,* published in 1771, contains vivid descriptions of what then was regarded as cancer:

> Cancer is either occult or manifest. An occult begins as a small indolent tumor about the size of a pea or hazelnut and may remain dormant for years. As soon as the virulent humor becomes more active, it begins to eat and break through the skin. Further occult cancers communicating with the glands arise afterwards. The parts being thus eaten away and consumed, death ensues.

> . . . a small, incipient, free cancer, seated in a suitable place, should be extirpated without delay, for unless it is extirpated root, branch, and feed, it will be exasperated and strike inwards, generate others and increase those already formed.[6:59]

The concept of cancer as a disease that eats and consumes is very old indeed.

The Parasitic Theory of Cancer

Although the parasitic theory of cancer was abandoned years ago, it continues to influence strongly psychosocial reactions to the disease.[3,5,8] In the seventeenth and eighteenth centuries, cancer was considered to be slightly contagious. The first cancer hospital, La Lutte Contre le Cancer of Rheims, France, established in 1740 by Jean Godinot, was forced to move from the city in 1779 because of the strong fear of contagion by the city's inhabitants. With the development of microbiology in the nineteenth century, each newly discovered microorganism was implicated as a possible cause of cancer.

The feeling that cancer was contagious, along with the belief that cancer was incurable, created a leprosylike aura about the disease. With this came a sense of shame and horror and the stigmatization of the cancer patient. The parasitic theory is largely responsible for shaping public attitudes toward cancer—attitudes that still persist.

Existential Aspects

The Denial of Death

> My heart is sore pained within me; and the terrors of death are fallen upon me. Fearfulness and trembling are come upon me, and horror hath overwhelmed. [Psalm 55:4,5]

The heading of this section is the title of the 1974 Pulitzer Prize-winning book, *The Denial of Death,* by Ernest Becker.[9] In this author's opinion, Becker's book may well be one of the most profound works ever written. It is not a text on death and dying as the name implies, but an attempt to understand the psychodynamics of human behavior based upon the premise that an individual's greatest anxiety is the fear of death. An understanding of this concept is fundamental to an understanding of the dynamics of the behavior of individuals confronting cancer, since many will have a crisis of "being" or "existence." As Becker wrote, "The idea of death, the fear of it, haunts the human animal like nothing else; it is a mainspring of human activity—activity designed largely to avoid the fatality of death, to overcome it by denying in some way that it is the final destiny of man."[9:27]

Freud believed that personal death had no representation in the unconscious mind: "At the bottom no one believes in his own death ... in his unconscious, everyone of us is convinced of his own immortality."[10:27] Yet we are all too aware of the existential contradiction; that is, we have a transcendent mind capable of abstract analytical thought, but we are trapped in a body that will age, deteriorate, bleed, and ultimately die. Everything that humanity does is an attempt to deny and overcome this fate. We are aware of our importance and uniqueness, and at the same time we know that we will go back into the ground to rot. We hope and believe that the things we create are of lasting worth and meaning, that they will outlive death and decay, and that they are religious and heroic.

In order to function in everyday life, we cannot be aware constantly of the existential dilemma. We must deny or suppress it. We function in an everyday layer of glib, empty talk, clichés, and role-playing, tranquilized by the trivial. Although full humanness means full fear and trembling at least for some part of the waking day, it is impossible to stand up to the terror of one's condition without extreme anxiety. The human desires to be a god with the equipment of an animal, so he thrives on fantasies, "and perhaps no one notices that in a deeper sense he lacks a self."[9:150] Humanity needs pageants, gods, crowds, and special days to give form and body to the internal fantasy that we are immortal. In modern times, however, we have been disinherited by our own analytic strength, with which we have banished mystery, naive belief, and simpleminded hope. The level of illusion we live with will determine how much freedom, hope, and dignity we are allowed.

> The syllogism he had learned from Kiezewetter's logic: "Caius is a man, men are mortal, therefore Caius is mortal" always seemed to him correct as applied to Caius, but certainly not as applied to himself. That Caius—man in the abstract—was mortal was perfectly correct, but he was not Caius, not an abstract man, but a creature quite, quite separate from all others. [Tolstoy: *The Death of Ivan Ilyich*]

Confrontation with cancer makes the denial of death, or at least the denial of the possibility of dying, no longer possible. As one patient said, "Having cancer is the embodiment of the existential paradox."[11] The first reaction to the realization that the disease may be malignant begins "when the icy fingers of contemplated death touch him."[12] Once the suspicion of having cancer is aroused, the patient will analyze everything said by the physician, intern, or nurse in an attempt to find out if the remarks or tone indicate a good or bad omen. This suspicion is based on fear, and fear in turn increases the suspicion. This fear is more than just a fear of death, but includes the fear of mutilation from treatment, the fear of pain, and the fear of loss of dignity.

In terms of the existential dualism, a confrontation with cancer makes the denial of death no longer possible. The individual stands stark naked, unprotected from the terror of his own death and decay. He seems unprotected from absolute oblivion.

Death is the "obscene mystery," the ultimate affront, the event that cannot be controlled but can only be denied.[1] The postponement of death is not the solution to the fear of death, since there still remains a fear of eventually dying. In clinical oncology this is best exemplified by the adult patient with acute leukemia whose disease is temporarily in remission. This is one of the most unique circumstances in all of medicine. In this situation all evidence of disease has been suppressed. The blood, bone marrow, and apparent physical health have returned to normal, yet the disease in all likelihood will recur and the patient will die—in six months, 12 months, two years, or five years—but eventually the patient will die from recurrence of leukemia. How do individuals cope during remission with the awareness that their death is imminent? The authors evaluated a small group of adult acute leukemia patients who were in remission.[13] Although our research is currently incomplete, it seems that denial is the most significant single defense mechanism, denial of illness, denial of the possibility of relapse, and denial of death from the disease. It seems that once the initial shock and initial therapy have passed, some patients are capable of reconstructing every effective denial mechanism, even the denial of death, in the face of what may seem an impossible situation.

Theological Aspects

> "My God, my God, why hast thou forsaken me?" [Psalm 22:1, Matthew 27:46, Mark 15:34]

Many powerful emotions have been and continue to be expressed in a religious context. This is especially true with regard to the reactions of an individual confronting cancer. There are many very basic theological issues she must face: (1) her personal concept of immortality, (2) her concept of the role of the church, (3) her concept of cancer as perhaps representing punishment, and (4) if she does believe her cancer represents punishment, what has she done to deserve it?

According to Sevensky,[14] religion serves at least three functions for the sick or dying patient. First, it provides a theoretical framework with which to make some sense of illness and mortality, for example, understanding them in terms of punishment, education, purification, sacrifice, or mystery. Religion allows a context without denying the reality of these experiences. Second, it provides practical resources for coping with illness, suffering, and mortality, including social support and ritual actions aimed at forgiveness, transcendence, and healing. Third, religion gives hope in the face of inevitable death. The idea that suffering has something valuable to teach us about reality and about ourselves is a theme found in all world religions. The hope that there is some lesson to be learned has sustained many who are faced with what otherwise would appear to be a hopeless, absurd, and empty experience. "In the face of all the odds against us, we build cathedrals . . . we pray for our immortal souls."[15]

The cancer patient may interpret suffering as in some sense sacrificial. Sacrifice in turn might support the hope of immortality.[16] The concept that we might leave this world without consequence is a thought which may be intolerable. Oblivion is incomprehensible. We each, therefore, have some concept of immortality, which may fit within the context of an organized religion or may reflect a more individual, idiosyncratic interpretation.

According to Weisman,[17] most religious viewpoints are based upon one of the following versions of death and, by implication, immortality:

1. *Metamorphosis:* the belief in rebirth following physical death, but without consciousness of a previous existence.
2. *Restoration:* the view that another life follows death, but one in which recollection is retained.
3. *Extinction:* the concept that there is no knowledge of anything beyond the grave, but personal continuity is guaranteed by means of good works, exemplary behavior, ethical standards, and so on.

In each conception of death some token evidence of our life testifies to our abiding presence and assures our continuity.

To many individuals the standard theological concept of immortality are unacceptable. For example, an artist or a genius in any given area earns his value as a person by means of his creativeness. His work justifies his existence and transcends death by qualifying him for immortality. He therefore creates his own immortality.[9] Freud stated, "Immortality means being loved by many anonymous people . . . living in the esteem of men yet unborn."[10] But it is hard to work steadfastly when your work may "mean no more than the cries of dinosaurs."[9]

According to Otto Rank,[18] the human is a theological being as well as a biological one. Rank noted our need for a sense of "symbolic immortality." He believed that science abandoned the word "soul" for the word "self" in order to make the mysteries of life and death subject to the laws of determinism.

> It seems to be difficult for the individual to realize that there exists a division between one's spiritual and purely human needs, and that the satisfaction of fulfillment for each has to be found in different spheres. As a rule, we find the two aspects hopelessly confused in modern relationships, where one person is made the god-like judge over good and bad in the other person. In the long run, such a symbiotic relationship becomes demoralizing to both parties, for it is just as unbearable to be God as it is to remain an utter slave.[18:138]

The cancer patient is confronted with the probability of his own personal death, a death that he can no longer deny. He must for the first time question the adequacy of his concept of immortality. He must question the very significance of his existence. He must question the possibility of oblivion.

> When I thought to know this,
> it was too painful for me.
>   [Psalm 73:16]

Anticipatory Grief

> A grief without a pang, void, dark and drear,
> A stifled, drowsy, unimpassioned grief,
> Which finds no natural outlet, no relief;
> In a word, or sigh, or tear
>   [Samuel Taylor Coleridge, "Dejection, An Ode"]

In a confrontation with a life-threatening illness such as cancer, death is perceived as a possible outcome. In this sense, life-threatening illness differs from terminal illness qualitatively and/or quantitatively. After an initial period of extreme psychological turmoil expressed as shock, anger, depression, and denial, the individual experiences a profound sense of grief or, more accurately, anticipatory grief.[19] He grieves for his own death from cancer. He grieves for the possibility of his death from surgery. He grieves because of possible disfigurement and permanent change of his body image. He grieves for potential loss of sexual function and physical attractiveness. He grieves because there may need to be an alteration in a basic bodily function, such as a colostomy.[20] He grieves because of the risk of permanent separation from family, loved ones, professional associates, pets, property. He grieves for the threatened loss of everything he has ever known, possessed, or loved, and the grief is accentuated by uncertainty.

The whole issue of uncertainty is one of the most difficult problems precipitated by the confrontation with a life-threatening illness.[21] Initially, the uncertainty surrounds the diagnosis: Are the symptoms those of an occult malignancy? Anxiety increases progressively and culminates when the diagnosis is confirmed. The next uncertainty concerns the outcome of the treatment: Will the surgery or radiation therapy or chemotherapy be successful? Following initial therapy, uncertainty evolves around the significance of minor symptoms: Does pain in the abdomen, or back, or chest mean the cancer is recurring? Following documented recurrence, uncertainty again becomes a significant issue: Will the second attempt at cure be successful? Does anyone really get a second chance? How much time do I have? Will there be pain? In the face of extreme pain, can I maintain my dignity as a human being?

Confrontation with a life-threatening illness is a "no-exit"[22] situation. No quantity of wealth, personal power, or influence can alter the reality of cancer. Nothing can protect one from the terror, the fear, the doubt, the suspicion, the loneliness, the isolation. Everyone is alone with this uncertainty and anxiety. Everyone is alone with his cancer.

Learned Helplessness

Approximately 10 years ago, the experimental psychologist Martin E.P. Seligman[23,24] described the phenomenon of learned helplessness in laboratory animals. The learned helplessness concept partly explains why some individuals are completely unable to cope with life-threatening diseases such as cancer. Simply put, these individuals, like Seligman's laboratory animals, have learned to accept themselves as helpless in all stressful situations because, at some earlier time, they were faced with severe trauma over which they had no control and from which they could not escape. Seligman's experiments showed that previous experience with uncontrollable trauma typically has three basic effects on animals: (1) they become passive in the face of trauma, (2) those who have become "helpless" will be retarded in learning that their responses can control trauma, and (3) they show more stress when faced with trauma they cannot control than with equivalent controllable trauma.

Seligman extends his hypothesis to human behavior, particularly reactive depression, which he feels has a number of parallels to the phenomenon of learned helplessness. He also applies this hypothesis to "voodoo deaths," first observed and documented by the American physiologist, W.B. Cannon,[25,26] who noted how members of various primitive cultures would die within hours of being cursed by a ritual gesture of a witch doctor or shortly after discovering that something they did previously broke a taboo.

G.W. Milton[27] has described a phenomenon in cancer patients which he feels is analogous to the voodoo deaths in primitive peoples. He reports that there does exist a small (and we emphasize *small*) group of patients in whom the realization of impending death is a blow so terrible that they are quite unable to adjust to it and they die rapidly, before the malignancy seems to have developed enough to cause death. Typically, this will be the response of a big man who is proud of his virility. The patient, when first confronted with the problem of malignant disease, appears to disregard it and may appear to be extraordinarily cheerful. Overnight the patient's whole manner changes. He literally turns his face to the wall and lies inert in bed, covering his face with the bedclothes. Within a month of the onset of this syndrome, the patient almost certainly will be dead. To continue the parallel, primitive people feel that a more powerful witch doctor may be able to overcome the curse of his rival; likewise, according to Milton, a cancer patient experiencing this syndrome may have a dramatic reversal if sent to a highly specialized cancer clinic. That is, as soon as he feels something can be done to help him, his mental attitude, and possibly physical condition, will improve.

> Do not go gentle into that good night,
> Rage, rage against the dying of the light.
> [Dylan Thomas]

Optimism and Hope

Optimism and hope are central to human life.[28] We all share a hopeful recognition of the future's promise. The anticipated growth of children, zest for sexual pleasure, appetite for strawberry shortcake, and buying two tubes of toothpaste are all actions that reflect a benign sense of the future. This sort of future is one in which the individual exerts control, is socially desirable, and finds living to be worthwhile and pleasurable. Anticipating optimistic outcomes for uncertain situations is a central and unique characteristic of human nature. We all share a fundamental optimism about the next moment, the next meal, the next day. In short, our sense of the future is more than just benign; we look forward to it; we are future oriented.

A confrontation with cancer severely alters one's orientation toward the future and may convert it to abject futurelessness. This is illustrated in a somewhat flippant comment made by a professional colleague who had had a melanoma removed from his shoulder one and one-half years previously: "I had always thought that if you had a melanoma you didn't go out and buy any more long-playing records."

Loss of future orientation is equivalent to loss of hope. Hope preserves dignity. Hope reinforces denial, and, as Becker wrote, "without possibility [hope] a man cannot, as it were, draw breath."[9:207]

As a rule patients with advanced cancer often consent to participation as experimental subjects in clinical trials evaluating new chemotherapeutic agents. Several years ago we attempted to evaluate this phenomenon by interviewing 50 consecutive patients with advanced cancer who were being treated on cooperative group chemotherapy protocol studies evaluating new agents.[29,30] The motivations of this entire group of 50 patients were indeed complex, and seldom if ever did individual patients state only a single reason for volunteering for investigational chemotherapy. They all expressed that the investigational treatment offered them greater *hope* than standard therapy. They hoped for increased chances of survival and relief of pain. Over half of the patients (29 out of 50) also expressed altruistic reasons for volunteering. These patients developed a sense of commitment to a cause and their morale improved even if their disease did not. Their cancer was no longer a cloaked executioner; rather, it was their adversary and they were joining forces with clinical investigators in an attempt to find a cure. The clinical research program had given their lives new meaning. And finally, patients volunteered because of physician trust: "The doctor wouldn't suggest it unless he thought it would help." "Doctors do not jeopardize their patients."

Freireich,[31] in a discussion of ethical considerations in cancer chemotherapy, has arrived at essentially the same conclusion regarding the role of clinical research as a means of psychological support for the patient with advanced cancer. An effective treatment for hopelessness is legitimate scientific research. Research offers hope of real benefit. The patient should have the potential for benefits emphasized so that he can receive the emotional support that research offers. Effective new treatments have emerged, and, while the frequency of benefits are often less than the frequency of failure, experimental chemotherapy offers the patient a significant alternative. In the Phase I (new experimental drug) study, the hope that cancer chemotherapy gives the patient far outweighs the side-effects of therapy. Participation in good clinical research may be one of the most effective psychological support systems available to the cancer patient, and one of the most effective buffers in the patient's confrontation with cancer.

Synthesis

Confrontation with cancer makes it impossible to continue to deny the fact that we ourselves eventually will die. Our concept of our own individual immortality is stressed to its limit. Our façade, the pretense that we have a degree of immortality not granted to anyone else, is ripped to the ground.

How we react to this confrontation will determine how well we can accept cancer patienthood. Will we become helpless, incapable of comprehending that help is available? Will we react to cancer as if a curse has been placed upon us, lying down to die as primitive people do when a witch doctor curses them? Will we grieve over the potential or actual changes in our body function or body image to the extent that we are incapable of adapting? Will the periods of uncertainty be too difficult to allow us to cope?

Despite the terrors of cancer, most people are able to maintain the optimism and hope characteristic of the human animal. This hope can be enhanced by the involvement of the patients in the decision-making process regarding their therapy. This allows them a sense of control over their destiny and helps combat the hopelessness, helplessness, and powerlessness associated with the loss of good health.

Finally, participation in clinical research trials not only affords some patients a means of psychological support, but also can provide good medical therapy for advanced cancer, otherwise unavailable. The cancer patient who participates in the clinical research program can develop a greater sense of hope, purpose, and commitment.

A confrontation with cancer can be devastating to the patient, physically, psychologically, and theologically. Understanding these aspects of the disease is fundamental to cancer medicine.

References

1. Sontag S: *Illness as Metaphor.* New York, Farrar Straus and Giroux, 1977.
2. Breasted JH: *The Edwin Smith Papyrus.* Chicago, University of Chicago Press, 1930, pp 403–406.
3. Kadinal CG, Yarbro JW: A conceptual history of cancer. *Seminars in Oncology* 6:396–408, 1979.
4. King LS: *The Philosophy of Medicine: The Early Eighteenth Century.* Cambridge, Mass., Harvard University Press, 1978.
5. Kardinal CG: An outline of the history of cancer. Parts I, II, and III. *Missouri Medicine* 74:662–664, 1977; 75:10–14, 74–78, 1978.
6. *Encyclopaedia Brittanica,* ed 1, vol II, p 18; vol III, pp 59, 139–140, 167, 664. Edinburgh, Scotland, William Benton, 1771.
7. Shimkin MB: *Contrary to Nature,* DHEW publication No. (NIH) 76-720. Washington, D.C., U.S. Government Printing Office, 1977.
8. Cassileth BR: The evolution of oncology as a sociomedical phenomenon, in BR Casileth (ed), *The Cancer Patient: Social and Medical Aspects of Care.* Philadelphia, Lea and Febiger, 1979.
9. Becker E: *The Denial of Death.* New York, The Free Press, 1973.
10. Freud S: *Thoughts for the Times: On War and Death.* London, The Hogarth Press, 1957, Vol XIV.
11. Trillon AS: Of dragons and garden peas: A cancer patient talks to doctors. *New Engl J Med* 304:699–701, 1981.
12. Milton GW: Thoughts in the mind of a person with cancer. *Br Med J* 4:221–223, 1973.
13. Sanders JB, Kardinal CG: Adaptive coping mechanisms in adult acute leukemia patients in remission. *JAMA* 238:952–954, 1977.
14. Sevensky RL: Religion and illness: An outline of their relationship. *South Med J* 74:745–750, 1981.
15. Tiger L: Optimism: The biological roots of hope. *Psychology Today* 12(1): 18–33, 1979.

16. Bakan D: *Disease, Pain, and Sacrifice: Toward a Psychology of Suffering.* Boston, Beacon Press, 1971.
17. Weisman AD: *On Dying and Denying: A Psychiatric Study of Terminality.* New York, Behavioral Publications, 1972.
18. Rank O: *Beyond Psychology.* New York, Dover Books, 1958.
19. Gullo SV, Cherico DJ, Sjadick R: Suggested stages and response styles in life-threatening illness: A focus on the cancer patient, in Schoenberg B, Carr AC, Kutscher AH, Peretz D, Goldberg I (eds), *Anticipatory Grief.* New York and London, Columbia University Press, 1974.
20. Rush BF Jr: A surgical oncologist's observations, in Schoenberg B, Carr AC, Kutscher AH, Peretz D, Goldberg I (eds), *Anticipatory Grief.* New York and London, Columbia University Press, 1974.
21. Kardinal CG, Sanders JB: The impact of cancer. *Forum on Medicine* 2: 603–607, 1979.
22. Sartre JP: *No Exit and Three Other Plays.* New York, Random House, 1955.
23. Seligman MEP: *Helplessness: On Depression, Development, and Death.* San Francisco, WH Freeman, 1975.
24. Seligman MEP: Learned helplessness. *Annual Review of Medicine* 23:407–412, 1972.
25. Cannon WB: "Voodoo" death. *American Anthropologist* 44:169–181, 1942.
26. Cannon WB: "Voodoo" death. *Psychosomatic Medicine* 19:182–190, 1957.
27. Milton GW: Self-willed death or the bone pointing syndrome. *Lancet* 1:1435–1436, 1973.
28. Tiger L: *Optimism: The Biology of Hope.* New York, Simon and Schuster, 1979.
29. Kardinal CG, Cupper HT: Reactions of patients with advanced cancer to their diagnosis and treatment. *Military Medicine* 142:374–376, 1977.
30. Kardinal CG, Cupper HT: Hope, consent, and clinical research. *Forum on Medicine* 1(8):48–49, 1979.
31. Freireich EJ: Ethical considerations in cancer chemotherapy. *Annual Review of Pharmacology and Toxicology* 19:547–557, 1979.

13

Psychosocial Problems and Communication in Terminal Care*

Barrie R. Cassileth and James Stinnett

The current discontent with the American health care system,[1] and probably the growing involvement of many patients with unorthodox therapies as well, stem in part from increased technologic advance resulting in highly specialized professional functions. This has led to narrowly defined clinical roles and to a common longing among patients for the less clinically sophisticated but more personally satisfying kind of doctor-patient relationship typical of past decades.

In many respects, "psychosocial support" is a modern euphemism for the qualities of human warmth, caring, and interpersonal skills characteristic of the bygone doctor-patient interaction. Nowhere is the patient's need for this kind of support more pressing than during terminal illness. Ironically, nowhere throughout the span of illness and treatment is that support less available from primary caregivers than during the terminal phase. Other professionals are available to deal with dying patients' psychological needs—psychiatrists, social workers, clergy, even thanatologists—and the temptation is great to call upon them, thereby to justify our decreasing contact as the patient slips clinically beyond capacity for therapeutic intervention.

The sense that true professionalism excludes emotional involvement, the perception that time and skills are more efficiently and effectively spent with aggressively-treatable patients, and the absence of training and guidelines for helpful interactions with dying patients leave us unarmed, unschooled, and uncomfortable. There is a large body of data, much of it based on solid studies

*This chapter was reproduced with permission of the publisher, from Cassileth, B.R., and Cassileth, P.A. (Eds.), *Clinical Care of the Terminal Cancer Patient*. Philadelphia, Lea & Febiger, 1982, chapter 8.

of terminally ill patients, which provides helpful information on the needs of such patients and on how clinicians can interact most beneficially.

This chapter is approached from a perspective involving three general premises. The first is that the business of *living,* of sustaining or enriching relationships, and of maximizing remaining time, is the proper focus of energies and goals for the terminal patient and for the clinician. The second is that dying is not a psychiatric disorder; that labels of psychologic dysfunction have little place or utility in the care of the terminally ill. The third is that the clinician's responsibility for the terminal patient includes psychosocial support; that such support is a legitimate and feasible portion of the physician's obligation.

A caveat is in order, however, with regard to the final premise. Although every patient requires and deserves the physician's continued support, not every patient requires special or additional intervention. Many people have the inner resources and family support not only to manage well on their own, but even to help others in the process. Many patients exhibit striking and surprising degrees of psychic strength and resourcefulness.

With today's emphasis on death and the current popularity of publications on the subject, the danger exists that an individual's behavior may be judged deficient or incorrect against some theoretical norm of what is "appropriate" or "healthy" during the final phase of life. The possibility of this danger is increased by overzealous interpretation of Elisabeth Kübler-Ross' analysis of the stages of death.[2] This pioneering work, despite the author's explicit warning, is readily perverted into the simplistic notion that people go neatly from one stage to another, and that anyone out of step requires psychological assistance. Not all patients experience particular stages of emotional response, and some remain comfortably fixed in a single emotional niche. It is the individual's own comfort, judged against a highly personalized standard, that must guide assessment. Whether an individual conforms to a general or idealized prototype of the "dying patient," if indeed one exists, is neither relevant nor helpful.

Communication

The area of communication exemplifies two extremes of a problem highlighted by the contemporary focus on death and dying. On the one hand, there is a tendency to expect and encourage all patients to verbalize their concerns and feelings about death; on the other, there is a preference among the more traditionally schooled to avoid any such discussion at all costs. Neither approach, indiscriminantly applied, can serve the best interests of patients.

The relatively nonverbal individual, the person whose feelings throughout life have remained matters of the utmost privacy, the intellectual who finds comfort in removing personal experience to a universal or literary plane, is treated inappropriately if pressed to discuss how "*you* feel about *your* impending death."[3] The other extreme tendency is perhaps more common: our frequent inability or unwillingness to admit to the patient that we know he is dying.

This may be the new conspiracy of silence. The issue is no longer whether to reveal a cancer diagnosis, but rather how to acknowledge to patients the sorrow and importance of their impending death. This is an aspect of communication difficult not only for clinicians, but for patients' friends and relatives as well. Forced to deal alone with the magnitude of their situation and with its terrible sadness, such patients are truly abandoned even in the midst of good clinical care and attentive family and staff. The conspiracy of silence denies patients the opportunity to ventilate and share concerns if they wish to do so. It cuts them off not only from meaningful communication with others, but also from the relief that the act of sharing one's concerns and feelings typically brings. This unwillingness or inability to talk about death, or to allow patients to do so, contributes to the fear of abandonment that, along with fears of pain, represent dying patients' most prevalent concerns.

Many find the subject of death uncomfortable because it is difficult to know what to say. We dread the "Why me?" questions that patients may ask, and we ourselves may harbor the same "Why this patient?" doubts. As clinicians, we are accustomed to ready answers, and here there are none at all. What dying patients need and want from us, however, are not answers but concern and interest. The challenge is less what to say than how to listen.

There are some specific points of explanation and reassurance that many patients welcome. Patients need to be assured of their physician's continuing involvement and participation in their care. The dying patient, moved to a room at the end of the hospital corridor and visited by staff with decreasing frequency and for ever shorter periods of time, is by now apocryphal, but remains a persistent reality in many instances.

The explicit statement that pain will be monitored and controlled continuously, accompanied of course by action toward that promise, is profoundly relieving to patients who have long-standing memories of the agonies of a dying relative years ago, or whose primary association with terminal cancer is lingering, painful death. Few patients ask directly, but many worry privately about the specifics of how they will die. One patient with leukemia, then at home, carried for months the fear that his death would occur suddenly, possibly while driving his wife and children in their car, and that he would destroy his entire family as a result of his own sudden death. He was greatly relieved to learn that death would occur gradually, and that adequate time would be available to prepare and protect his family.

Patients and families are reassured also to learn that death, almost invariably, is preceded by gradual loss of function and by peace and tranquility. It is devoid of fear or anguish, an observation made by Osler and many others.[4,5] Many fear suffocation, a realistic concern about a problem that can be managed. Other patients have expressed the irrational fear that, while receiving palliative radiation therapy, the radiation apparatus might fall on them or that no one would know if they were in distress and in need of help.

Patients often harbor frightening fantasies, such as that of sudden death, which are readily correctable. Fantasies and similar concerns can be handled, but only if we know what they are. Knowing requires giving patients the opportunity to talk and to voice their worries, which in turn requires our willingness to be there and listen.

Alienation and Loss of Control

The almost total dependency of the hospitalized terminally ill patient is a source of frustration and humiliation, particularly for those whose lives have been characterized by independence and decision making for self and others. Hospitalization, even for short-term, minor ailments is associated with anxiety, depersonalization, loss of control, and the disquiet induced by unintelligible terminology used in reference to oneself.

All of these problems are exacerbated for terminally ill patients who also face a childlike existence in which physical needs are attended to by others, in which relief from pain and discomfort depend upon people and actions outside of themselves, and in which progressive debilitation increasingly narrows their sphere of independent capacity and action. In part, appeals for "death with dignity" and "quality of remaining life," as well as the popularity of hospice facilities, are attributable directly to these unfortunate circumstances of terminal hospitalization.

The sense of alienation and loss of control can be decreased at least to a degree, but usually at some cost to the efficiency of hospital routine. Patients should be given the opportunity to make decisions whenever possible. In the absence of therapeutic preference, the option to receive medication in liquid versus capsule form, for example, should be offered the patient. Patients should be given the opportunity to medicate themselves where feasible and should have copies of their own medication schedules. Whenever possible, self-care and the opportunity to select preferred menus also will help the patient regain some control over the environment and the disease. Removing from a patient all opportunity to act independently defeats the goal of enabling patients to maximize their remaining time and to "live" until they die. The patient who is rendered totally dependent to suit institutional needs is socially "dead" before his time.

Types of Death

Pattison[6] delineates four definitions of death, a conceptualization that is clinically useful as well as theoretically interesting. The first is "sociologic death," the withdrawal and separation from the patient by others. Depending on the patient's physical environment and the reactions of family and staff, sociologic death can last for days or weeks if the patient is left alone to die; for years if the patient has been abandoned, unvisited, in a nursing home; or for minutes if the patient remains surrounded by caring others until the moment of actual death.

The second type is "psychic death," in which patients accept death as imminent and regress into themselves. Usually psychic and actual death occur almost simultaneously, but some patients give up, accept death prematurely, and refuse to continue living.

"Biologic death," the third type, is defined as the absence of cognitive function or awareness, although artificial support systems may sustain vital organ functioning.

Fourth is "physiologic death," wherein all vital organs have ceased to function.

The ordinary sequence of events proceeds from sociologic through physiologic death, but distortions of this process can occur. Inappropriately early sociologic death, for example, is a common phenomenon when patients are abandoned or when family members, given a projected length of survival, find the patient still alive months after the expected time limit has elapsed. This problem can be precluded by avoiding specific projections of survival time, such as, "He has approximately four months to live." "Psychic" death can occur prematurely for patients who view a cancer diagnosis as stigmatizing and tanamount to immediate demise. If recognized, such emotional reactions are reversible.

Guilt

Adults as well as children may interpret terminal illness, particularly terminal malignant disease, as punishment for past failures or actions. The impact of this kind of thinking has been magnified in recent years by popularization of the notion that maintaining and regaining health are primarily responsibilities of the individual. Although there is validity in the concept that we are responsible for certain behaviors that carry health risks, such as smoking, poor diet, and lack of exercise, the popularized notion unfortunately also embodies the precept that one is at fault personally not only for having contracted cancer, but also for the failure to achieve cure.

A school teacher with metastatic melanoma requested a psychotherapeutic interview. She had a single, straightforward question: "Did I do this to myself by working too hard for the past 10 years?" Her question received an emphatic no. Demonstrably relieved, she was unburdened of massive guilt carried secretly since her diagnosis some months before. The guilt had been inspired by a newspaper article sponsoring the view that all illness is self-inflicted and that cancer is incurable only if one strives inadequately or ineffectively to overcome it.

Psychosocial factors no doubt contribute in an as-yet-unknown manner to the etiology of disease, but only as one link in a very long causal chain. The direct relationship, postulated by some, that emotional deficit or improper lifestyle cause malignant disease, is untenable. Worse, it adds the burden of guilt to the patient already struggling with the physical and emotional difficulties of terminal illness.

Alternative Cancer Therapies

The natural corollary to the notion that cancer is caused by psychosocial factors is that cancer can be cured through the patient's mental and physical efforts. This has resulted in the use of mind-control, dietary, and internal cleanliness efforts to treat cancer, which are characteristic of alternative cancer treatments today. It is of interest that current unorthodox therapies differ substantially from alternative remedies offered throughout the past century. Previous unorthodox treatments were "medicines," or at least "medicinal." They came in ampules, vials, or syringes; they were visual duplicates of standard medications, administered in the usual clinical fashion and sold by people in white coats.

Today's alternative remedies implicitly and explicitly reject any association with standard treatment. Proponents emphasize the distinction and distance of these remedies from anything medical. These are "antimedicines." The new alternative therapies involve no agents requiring FDA approval; they emphasize dietary proscription and recommendation and involve procedures and techniques that can be self-administered or handled by people with no particular training. These therapies, therefore, cannot be categorized as quasi- or illegitimately medical, but rather as aspects of lifestyle, beyond licensing or regulation.

It is no coincidence that the alternative cancer treatments popular today reflect an antimedicine, pro-self-help bias. Acceptance of contemporary unorthodox approaches occurs in the context of an increasingly depersonalized and unsatisfying health care system and during a period of mounting public distrust of a medical establishment that has failed to find a cure for cancer, despite substantial time and financial support.

Two important deficiencies in the traditional system, deficiencies that deeply concern cancer patients, represent the core of the alternative therapy approach: (1) personalized interest in the patient as a person and (2) the patients' self-involvement or control over their disease. Patients receiving alternative treatments are required to maintain responsibility for their own care through exquisitely detailed and highly specialized dietary regimens, internal cleansing techniques, and/or mental exercises; and they receive from their alternative therapists the kind of whole-patient concern that they find missing in the traditional doctor-patient relationship.

Coping

Our ability to help patients cope demands just those qualities that patients find wanting in the traditional medical setting, and that they find more readily available from alternative therapists. The capacity to sit and listen runs contrary to our activist, interventionist orientation. The simple act of sitting down with a patient carries important meaning: It suggests a willingness and readiness for real communication. But clinicians typically stand at the bedside, and this posture itself conveys a message that is rarely misinterpreted. The patient knows that the physician is too busy with more important matters to sit down and talk. It is a unique patient who can share concerns in a meaningful and productive fashion with an individual looming over the bed, demonstrating by posture the hope and expectation of a quick departure.

Patients' needs differ from one day to the next, and each patient is unlike the other. Helpful interaction requires some understanding of the emotional status and needs of a particular patient at that point in time, understanding that can be achieved by a willingness to listen and to confront issues that are as difficult for the physician as for the patient.

The terminal patient faces a crisis of major proportions and the overwhelming prospect of extinction. It is a natural survival technique for all of us under conditions of great stress to segment the overall problem or task and to deal with smaller, more manageable pieces of the whole on a sequential basis. Our approach to terminal patients can help them similarly to deal with manageable segments of the whole. We can guide them through incremental disappointments, each of which can be mastered before the next problem is confronted. Patients can be helped to avoid the need to face one massive loss by the manner and timing of our presentation of information. The opportunity for time during which adjustment to incremental loss may occur is important and needed. We can be guided successfully by the assessment of how much this patient is ready to be told at this particular point and by knowledge of where the patient is in the continuum of adjustment to incremental disappointment. The goal is to obviate the patient's need to confront the totality of the loss all at once.

Patients readjust their self-perceptions and goals according to their changing clinical status. It is often difficult for the healthy outsider to understand how and where terminal patients find reason for hope or for the setting of goals. Patients do, however, reorient themselves and establish goals—such as going home, or living long enough to attend an anniversary—that are consonant with their physical realities.

Denying or minimizing the seriousness of the situation is a common and adaptive coping mechanism that also gives patients time to assimilate the impact of the sequential implications of their illness. Temporary denial affords the opportunity to marshall psychologic resources needed to deal with the problem. Temporary denial among seriously ill patients is not psychopathologic; it serves a useful and adaptive purpose by buffering the impact of new realities. Denial serves the important purpose discussed previously: It gives patients time to cope with small setbacks, rather than having to face the problem in its entirety at one time, and it should not be interfered with. House staff occasionally are alarmed by patients who they conclude are doing poorly because they "won't talk about their dying." Not all patients talk about their dying when one might think they should, and some patients never verbalize the subject. If the mechanism of denial makes the patient more comfortable and does not interfere with care, it should be respected and left alone. The well-meaning bias to help the patient "confront reality" should not be used as a rationale to batter successful adaptive defenses.

Anger is a natural response to massive disappointment and impending loss. Because it is difficult for rational people to display anger at something as inexplicable and abstract as fate or terminal disease, anger tends to be displaced onto potentially more controllable concrete or neutral aspects of the patient's environment, such as caregivers, hospital food or routine, or family members. We need to respond to patients' anger, but to its real rather than superficial meaning. Assaults should not be taken personally, nor dealt with at face value. Instead of reacting to the patient's words by, for example, apologizing for inadequately hot food, a more helpful response would confront the source of the anger ("I know you're angry. It's awful to be so sick and I feel terrible about it too.") Anger is another coping response which helps the patient gain mastery and control over an essentially uncontrollable situation.

Another type of effort to attain mastery is the attempt to find purpose or meaning in the illness and impending death. The meaning may be perceived in terms of religious faith or some other highly personal construct. If the ascribed meaning is detrimental, for example, if it involves guilt or self-blame for the disease, efforts on the part of the clinician and possibly outside intervention are needed to reorient the patient to a more reasonable and comfortable perspective. Typically, however, patients find purpose or meaning in their suffering in such a way as to provide spiritual or emotional relief, and they should be supported toward this goal.

Important individual differences color patients' needs and reactions. Cultural and situational factors modify pain thresholds, pain perception, and need for analgesics. The symbolic implications of cancer influence the meaning ascribed to the disease, readiness to comply with therapeutic regimens, and general emotional response.[7] Family support and demands, personality, lifestyle and internal resources, and habitual modes of coping with crisis help determine the quality of adaptation, the effectiveness of coping, the need for intervention, and the type of preferred doctor-patient relationship. Patients vary in their preference for detailed information and in the extent to which they want to participate in treatment decisions.[8]

It is clear that the needs and strengths of terminally ill patients are diverse. As such, each patient must be approached not according to some predetermined notion of "correct" attitudes and behavior, but rather through sensitivity to the unique qualities of the particular individual. In addition to variation across individuals, there is substantial variability over time within an individual patient with regard to needs and emotional status. Fluctuations are to be expected. A standard or uniform approach to patients, or even to a single patient across time, is no more appropriate than would be an invariate style of communication with one's colleagues or family.

Understanding what the patient is experiencing and serving that patient well demand professional role flexibility: emotional accessibility, the capacity to listen, and a readiness to share and thereby to help diminish grief. These are skills that we tend to have as individuals but are foreign to medical training and to our usual sense of what physicians should do and be. Of critical importance is that the patient's physician remain with the patient, continue to participate in management, and sustain contact throughout the terminal phase so that the patient's fears of abandonment will not be realized.

The patient's death is not our failure nor that of the medical system, and any guilt we may feel about an impending death is misplaced. Patients want and require of their physicians continued concern and attention. Patients assign blame and disappointment not to our inability to repel inevitable death, but to our discomfort and reluctance to share with them its tribulations and grief.

References

1. Knowles JH: Doing better and feeling worse: Health in the United States. *Daedalus* Winter:57, 1977.
2. Kübler-Ross E: *On Death and Dying.* New York, Macmillan, 1969.
3. Hudson RP: Death, dying, and the zealous phase. *Ann Intern Med* 88:696–702, 1978.
4. Parkes CM: Psychological aspects, in Garfield CA (ed): *Psychosocial Care of the Dying Patient.* New York, McGraw-Hill, 1978.
5. Thomas L: Notes of a biology watcher: The long habit. *New Engl J of Med* 286:825–826, 1972.

6. Pattison EM: The living–dying process, in Garfield CA (ed): *Psychosocial Care of the Dying Patient.* New York, McGraw-Hill, 1978.
7. Cassileth BR: The evolution of oncology as a sociomedical phenomenon, in Cassileth BR (ed): *The Cancer Patient: Social and Medical Aspects of Care.* Philadelphia, Lea & Febiger, 1979.
8. Cassileth BR, Zupkis RV, Sutton-Smith K, et al: Information and participation preferences among cancer patients. *Ann Intern Med* 92:832–836, 1980.

14

Toward a Behavioral Oncology

Thomas H. Budzynski and T. Flint Sparks

There are few instances in which the subjective warmth of humanism and the objective precision of science come together in such a synergistic way as in the treatment of a person suffering from an illness. The balance necessary for healing includes attention to the person—the individual—as well as to the disease from which that individual is suffering. This dynamic balance occurs not only interpersonally between the healer and the patient but may take place internally within the person in distress. In fact, some of the most potent forces guiding the healing process may come from deep within the patient and may be influenced, in part, by his or her beliefs (Frank, 1974).

These sorts of concepts are most readily observable in the treatment of psychosomatic diseases in which the interplay between the mind and body are seen most directly. And yet, the results of investigations into psychosomatic processes and psychophysiologic treatment modalities have begun to define features common to all natural healing processes mediated ultimately by the central nervous system. What has been seen most clearly in those special disease states we have labeled "psychosomatic" seems to occur in all states of health and illness. What has emerged is the notion that we as human beings are complex biopsychosocial systems that may operate in a regulated (i.e., healthy) fashion or become dysregulated to the point of symptom formation and clinical disease (Schwartz, 1979). So it is with cancer.

Merely observing the differences among people with cancer poses several interesting questions: Why do some patients respond quickly and positively to their treatments while other patients with the same diagnosis do poorly and die? Why, in very similar circumstances with almost identical exposure to cancer-causing agents, do some people develop a malignancy while others do not?

While there are no final answers to these questions as yet, there is mounting evidence that a number of factors, working together, may account for cancer development and progression and that psychological variables may weigh heavily among these factors.

In a comprehensive review, Sklar and Anisman (1981) state a similar perspective:

> Given the variability of cancer development among individuals exposed to similar amounts of carcinogens (see the review in Doll, 1977; . . . Nagao et al., 1978; Storer, 1975; Upton, 1975), it is tempting to speculate that besides environmental factors, psychological variables (e.g. coping, prior stress history) might contribute to the induction of tumors or the proliferation of cancer cells following carcinogen exposure.
>
> In addition to the effects of carcinogenic induction, it is conceivable that stress might influence the progress of the neoplasm in humans. [p. 394]

We feel that it is not only conceivable but likely that one's response to stress (one's coping style) may influence profoundly one's response to cancer and cancer treatments. We will offer a model that we believe integrates much of the relevant data from psychology, endocrinology, immunology, and oncology, data that address some of the perplexing questions drawn from our clinical observations. (See Sklar & Anisman, 1981, and Riley, 1981, for the most current and complete reviews in the field.)

Stress and Cancer Development

We use the term "stress" in a broad sense that includes any of the psychophysiological consequences of adaptation to change. In this way we account for the stressful aspects of seemingly positive change such as a business promotion or the beginning of a new and exciting love relationship, as well as for the more commonly thought of distressing results of a business or relationship failure. Despite our use of this definition in describing human stress, most of the animal studies that will be cited involve the use of aversive stimuli only.

The concept that stress may influence the onset or progression of a neoplasm is actually not a new idea. Studies begun in the 1940s were designed to identify correlations between stress and tumor growth. Reports at two major symposia on the psychophysiological aspects of cancer (New York Academy of Sciences, 1966, 1969) generally pointed toward a positive relationship; that is, as stress increases, tumors develop and grow faster. Then, as more studies using different tumor systems and different types of stress paradigms were used, conflicting reports began to emerge.

It appears that certain chronic physical stressors actually inhibited tumor incidence. Animals exposed to physical restraint (Newberry, Gildow, Wogan, & Reese, 1976), foot shock (Newberry, Frankie, Beatty, Maloney, & Gilchrist,

1972; Pradham & Ray, 1974; Ray & Pradham, 1974; Visintainer, Volpicelli, & Seligman, 1982), electroconvulsive shock and sound stress (Pradham & Ray, 1974) were observed to have reduced tumor incidence as compared with controls.

These data conflicted with results of other research and were made even more confusing by divergent results observed with different applications of the same stress. The timing of events in these experiments emerged as an important factor, and a crucial idea was discovered amid the confusing results. It appears that predictability of stress, a sort of expectation or anticipation of distress, is crucial in whether or not these chronic physical stressors inhibited or enhanced tumor incidence. Where there was physical stress alone, without warning, there was decreased tumor incidence. When the same physical stressor was signaled and therefore could be anticipated, there was higher incidence of tumors.

Stress and Tumor Growth

Experimental outcomes highlight the importance of the organism's ability to cope with stress so as to modulate the physical damage to the body. One of the most striking examples of this effect was demonstrated by Sklar and Anisman (1979) in an experiment in which mice were injected with P815 mastocytoma cells and were then exposed to either escapable or inescapable electrical shock. In this experiment the animals could either do something in response to their stress (get away) or could do nothing (remain in their restraints). The animals who could do nothing had tumors that appeared earlier and grew more rapidly than in those animals who could escape the shock. It appears that the ability to respond—something akin to coping in humans—was partially responsible for decreased tumor incidence and growth rates in the mice.

In these studies of tumor growth, the tumor-enhancing effects of social stress also were documented. It seems that social disturbance increases the growth of tumors in several animal systems (Dechambre & Gosse, 1973; Sklar & Anisman, 1980). Along with these confirmatory results were a series of studies that added an additional piece of information to the emerging understanding of stress and cancer. Several experiments such as the one previously described (Sklar & Anisman, 1979) all demonstrated that the pathological results of stress would be minimized if the animals in the experiments had the option of escaping from the stress (Anisman, Pizzino, & Sklar, 1980; Weiss, Glazer, & Pohorecky, 1976; Weiss, Stone, & Harrell, 1970). One such series of experiments demonstrated that fighting behaviors could in some way reduce the deleterious effects of stress (Amkraut & Solomon, 1972; Stolk, Conner, Levine, & Barchas, 1974; Weiss, Pohorecky, Salman, & Gruenthal, 1976). The work of Amkraut and Soloman specifically showed that fighting (a type of coping response) could not only reduce the neurochemical and ulcerative effects of stress as described by Selye (1956), but actually could reduce the incidence and growth rates of tumors in rats exposed to Maloney-murine sarcoma virus.

To this point, the data indicate that acute physical and either acute or chronic social stress increase the incidence of tumors and stimulate their growth rates in animal systems. In addition, we are beginning to see the importance of coping behaviors as powerful modulators of this tumorogenic effect.

Stress and Neuroendocrine Changes

The observation that increasing stress often is met with increasing incidence of cancer has been made for years. However, the mechanisms that mediate the links between stress and tumor incidence or growth have not been known and still are incompletely described. However, there are some clues within the central nervous system and its interactions with the endocrine and immune systems that offer some insights into possible mechanisms. In fact, there has been sufficient interest in the last few years in these processes to stimulate the entirely new field of "psychoimmunology" (Ader, 1981; Holden, 1980).

The experimental data documenting the pathological changes within the central nervous system and endocrine system as a result of stress are prodigious (see Selye, 1956; Riley, 1981; Sklar & Anisman, 1981). The studies all point to a central axis along which the deleterious effects of stress move. Generally, stress generates some cognitive/emotional stimulation within the brain's cortex. This cortical activity may send signals to lower structures, through the limbic system to the hypothalamus and pituitary and ultimately to the adrenal cortex. Adrenocortical activity results in increasing production and secretion of corticosterone. Increasing blood levels of corticosterone then may have marked effects on immune-system functioning as evidenced by lymphocytopenia (decrease in the number of circulating lymphocytes), thymus involution, and an atrophy of the spleen and lymph nodes (Riley, 1981). All of these changes, both endocrine and immune, can have direct effects on tumor induction and tumor growth (Furth, 1975; Huggins, 1967; Welsch & Nagasawa, 1977).

Although the axis just described seems to be a one-way chain of events, behavioral changes, which are ultimately central nervous system activities, can mediate the expression of this neurochemical process. Just as coping behaviors such as escape from shock limited the tumor-stimulating effects of that stressor in rats, escape from shock likewise limits the excess production and secretion of corticosterone (Weiss, 1971; Weiss, Glazer, & Pohorecky, 1976).

Within the brain itself, neurochemical changes occur as a result of stress (Anisman, 1978; Stone, 1975). Stress may contribute to the depletion of norepinephrine (Goldstein & Nakajima, 1966; Gordon, Spector, Sjoerdsma, & Udenfriend, 1966; Saarela, Hissa, Hohtola, & Jorenen, 1977; Simmonds, 1969) and of a number of other neurotransmitters such as acetylocholine, dopamine, and benzodiazepine receptors (Cherek, Lane, Freeman, & Smith, 1980).

In summary, it appears that stress causes alterations in the neurochemistry of the brain and in the levels of circulating corticosteroids in the blood. These changes in the brain and blood chemistry then affect the competence of the immune system. We know that stress may alter dramatically the incidence of cancer and the growth rate of animal tumors, and we know that the ability of the organism to cope with stress may diminish the pathological changes in all of these systems. These interactions are strongly suggestive of a neurochemical involvement in cancer growth and regression. The specific stress-related changes in the immune system will be elaborated further as a way of demonstrating the interactive nature of the brain, behavior, and physiology as related to cancer.

Stress and Immune-System Functioning

The crucial question in determining the influence of immunocompetence on tumor growth and development is whether or not the immune system actually influences tumor regression or progression. The assumption that the immune system is central to these processes is embodied in the immune surveillance hypothesis (Klein, 1973-74). However, direct evidence for such a process is incomplete at this time.

Despite the controversial nature of the immune surveillance hypothesis as a primary component in the development of cancer, it is clear that immunocompetence is an important factor in the *growth* of a malignancy and, hence, in the survival of the host. Therefore, an understanding of stress-related immune-system changes is important to a more complete understanding of cancer treatment. There are good reviews that summarize the work to date (see Amkraut & Solomon, 1975; Rogers, Dubey, & Reich, 1979).

Although there are no solid data that link behavioral response to stress and immunocompetence, two studies have shown that immunosuppression may be "behaviorally conditioned" (Ader & Cohen, 1975; Rogers et al., 1979). In these experiments animals were given cyclophosphamide (which is immunosuppressive) and saccharin, a sweet taste stimulus. After repeated pairing, immunosuppression could be seen in the experimental animals given saccharin alone. It is as if behavioral cues to stress, in this case taste, can generate physiological responses within the immune system.

If the competence of the immune system can be depressed with a simple conditioning paradigm and even more finely altered by varying the stressor, how much power might we ascribe to the effects of chronic disappointment, frustration, fear, or other complex emotional states in humans? This is an important issue that current research must address.

It is clear that results from a large number of studies from the field of immunology, endocrinology, neurology, psychology, and oncology interact in such a way as to provide new insights into the etiology and course of malignant diseases in animals. The next task is to determine to what extent these observations hold true for humans and what progress can be made in the management or prevention of malignancy. The essence of this task is stated clearly within the larger context of behavioral medicine by Gary Schwartz (1978):

> The extent to which the central nervous system is involved *functionally* in either "psychological" or "physical" disease is the extent to which psychosocial factors can play a role in the etiology and treatment of any disease. Interestingly, it is somewhat ironic that advances in the biological sciences currently provide the justification for *behavioral* intervention in health and disease. [p. 75]

With this as our position, we will offer a model with the brain as the central feature in understanding the psychoneuroimmune data already presented. However, it is worth reviewing first the data on stress and cancer in human populations as we move toward the description of a behavioral oncology.

Stress and Human Cancer

Although observations have been made and reports have appeared for many years linking emotional factors to cancer incidence and progression, only recently has research begun to demonstrate strong and consistent links among these factors (see Kissen, 1969; and LeShan, 1959, 1966, for historical reviews).

A great deal of research was begun in the 1950s and 1960s within the field of psychosomatic medicine in an attempt to define a "cancer personality," or a life-history pattern and subsequent behavior pattern that would predispose a person to the development of a malignancy. This personality typing approach was somewhat unsuccessful in terms of defining a set of clearly predictive criteria and has been reviewed critically by Fox (1978). This body of research was found to be unconvincing largely because the studies were either retrospective, did not include all the variables known to influence causation, or the instruments used in measuring stress or psychological factors were either invalid or unreliable. Fox's review was a crucial turning point in the field because it highlighted the lack of solid data and went on to define the reasons why the data were less than convincing, based on poor research design. Suggestions for future research were given, and new research has appeared. What is most interesting is that the new, well-developed research data seem to support the old results. What was suggested by early research is being "rediscovered" by more powerful designs.

The first prospective study to demonstrate a causative link between personality and disease was initiated in the 1940s by Thomas and Duszynski (1974). They interviewed and tested 1008 medical students and followed them for upwards of 30 years to determine if psychological factors would predict later physical illness. Within this group, 30 subjects developed cancer and were described as being people who perceived a lack of closeness to their parents as children. The result is interesting because it mirrors the results of previous work by Bahnson (1964), Kissen (1966), LeShan (1966), and Schmale and Iker (1966). All of these studies suggested that, along with lack of closeness to parents or other significant persons, loss and difficulty in communicating the emotional experiences of loss were central features in the psychological aspects of cancer development.

Horne and Picard (1979) followed up on this type of research by developing an experiment designed to determine psychosocial risk factors for lung cancer. In this study, 130 subjects were selected who had undiagnosed lung disease visible on x-ray examination. The subjects then participated in a semi-structured interview and completed a series of psychosocial scales. After assessment the medical diagnoses were assigned to the participants retrospectively. The psychosocial scale correctly predicted 80 percent of the individuals with benign disease and 61 percent of the individuals with malignant disease. What is interesting from an analysis of subscales was that the subscale called "Recent Significant Loss" was the best predictor of actual diagnosis. "Job Stability" and "Lack of Plans for the Future" also were instrumental in adding to the predictive nature of the psychosocial scale. These psychosocial data then were compared with the patients' smoking history as a predictor of malignant lung disease and the psychosocial factors were as much as *twice* as important in predicting the correct diagnosis.

These data, once again, point to the significance of loss as a predisposing factor in cancer development and demonstrate the potency of these factors when compared to the usual medical predictors such as smoking history in the etiology of lung cancer. However, this study was not entirely prospective, so further work is necessary to verify the results.

What often is implied in research that shows loss as a predisposing factor to illness is that the person experiences grief or depression in such a way that the psychophysiological components of their depression interact as part of the development of the malignancy. This implication was followed up by a group of researchers at Rush-Presbyterian-Saint Luke's Medical Center in Chicago. Bieliauskas and colleagues (Bieliauskas, Shekelle, Garron, Maliza, Ostfeld, Paul, & Raynor, 1979) gave the Minnesota Multiphasic Personality Inventory (MMPI) to 2020 men aged 40 to 55 in 1958. These men were followed carefully; by 1974, 83 of the men had died of cancer. When the scores on Scale 2 (D = Depression) of the MMPI for these 83 men were compared to the rest of the group, it was found that the Depression scale was significantly higher for the men who had died of cancer (p = .035). There were no significant differences on any of the other nine clinical scales. There were 379 men who had D as their highest scale score, and this group had twice the rate of death from cancer when compared to the remainder of the population. Interestingly, these differences in predictive odds for cancer death were not affected by adjustments made for age, cigarette smoking, or alcohol consumption. Once again, psychological factors—and the *same types* of psychological factors—emerge as predictive in cancer development.

If psychological factors weigh so heavily in cancer development, what evidence is there for a psychologically mediated effect on cancer progression or regression? In an experiment conducted by Derogatis, Abeloff, and Melisaratos (1979), women with metastatic breast cancer were interviewed, tested, and followed for two years. The women were separated into two groups at the end of that period. The short-term survivors had died within a year of their metastatic diagnosis. The long-term survivors had lived two years or more and passed their metastatic diagnosis. The authors described their results as follows:

> Clearly, the long-term survivors in this series manifested a psychological profile that suggests a characteristic response toward their illness . . . [They] appeared more capable of externalizing their negative feelings and aspects of the underlying conflicts that gave rise to them and did not appear to suffer any self-image loss as a result of communicating in this fashion. Patients who died more rapidly appeared distinctly less able to communicate dysphoric feelings—particularly those of anger and hostility—and their symptom profiles were not substantially different from normal. [p. 1507]

The importance of the ability to cope, whether it is escape from shock in animal systems or escape from the inner terror and anger of having cancer in humans, appears to be crucial in influencing survival times. And, once again, the predictive nature of the psychological variables was more powerful than age, menopausal status, sites of metastasis, or treatment received in determining survival times in this study. Similar results in a prospective study of breast cancer patients demonstrated that coping style was more powerful than most medical predictors in recurrence of early-stage breast cancer (Greer, 1979).

Research conducted at the National Cancer Institute by Rogentine and colleagues (Rogentine, Van Kammen, Fox, Docherty, Rosenblatt, Boyd, & Bunney, 1979) demonstrated the importance of coping in the relative rates of recurrence of malignant melanoma. In a two-part study the researchers tested 64 subjects with Stage I or II malignant melanoma, using a number of psychosocial instruments. One of these instruments was a scale that asked the patient to rate the amount of psychological adjustment required to cope with the illness. The scale ranged from 1 to 100, and subjects were asked to anticipate needing either a low degree of adjustment (a low score) or a high degree of adjustment (a high score). In the initial sample, 29 of the subjects had recurrent disease one year after surgery. Their scores were significantly *lower* on this scale than those of the nonrelapsers. These data were used in the second stage of the study to predict recurrence in the next 33 patients, who were matched according to disease severity with the first 69. The predictions were 70 percent accurate and were independent of known medical predictors of one-year survival.

Those patients who perceived the need for a high degree of adjustment and carried this out did better medically. These results are reminiscent of the experiments on animals who could either escape or not escape electric shock (Sklar & Anisman, 1979). Those organisms who do something in response to stress, whether it is escaping the shock or adapting to a serious illness, do better than those organisms who do or try nothing or very little. The neuroendocrine and immune-system data support this concept also. The animals that can fight are less susceptible to physical deterioration following stress than the animals that are more passive (e.g., Amkraut & Solomon, 1972). This is parallel to the data presented by Derogatis et al. (1979) and Greer et al. (1979). Results from those women who were fighters, expressed their emotions openly, or used some *active* means of coping, showed that either their cancer recurred less often or they survived their disease for longer periods.

The data with human subjects appear to fit a pattern similar to the one seen in animal studies. Although one cannot always compare animal and human data directly, the links are too close and the results of experiments are too consistent for us not to notice the patterns. As Vernon Riley (1981) has stated:

> Although it may be hazardous to extrapolate biological findings from mice to other species, it would be equally imprudent to ignore the many physiological similarities and analogous biochemical relationships that evolutionary biologists have demonstrated. [p. 1101]

The remaining factor discussed in the animal studies that only recently has been addressed with human subjects is the relationship between the brain and immunity as a possible mechanism in the growth of malignant tumors. No work has been done that conclusively links psychoimmune mechanisms to cancer, but there are data that suggest that emotional factors may influence immune-system functioning markedly in humans. Significant decreases in lymphocyte functioning have been recorded in subjects grieving over the loss of a spouse (Bartrop, Lazarus, Luckhurst, Kiloh, & Penny, 1977). *Loss* and the *ability to cope* have been shown repeatedly to influence both the onset and progression of neoplastic disease. This further tie to immune-system competence compels us to search for better understanding of the psychoneuroimmune factors in cancer development and treatment.

The next step in research is, of course, to apply the principles of the behavioral sciences in such a way as to enhance the behavior patterns that have been shown to correlate with better responses to cancer management. This is a complex task and has been approached systematically in only two pilot projects published to date (Gilbert, Miller, Gilbert, Budzynski, & Bernton, 1979; and Simonton, Matthews-Simonton, & Sparks, 1980). The results of these projects do suggest that psychological intervention as adjuncts to the standard treatment of a wide variety of cancers may be helpful to some patients, both emotionally and physiologically.

Stress Management in Cancer Patients

The accumulated results of studies such as those noted previously indicate that chronic, uncontrolled stress may lead to the development of cancer in certain individuals. This type of stress apparently weakens the body's immunological defenses. In cancer patients the immune system may be weakened further by the very same treatment procedures (surgery, radiation, and chemotherapy) that are directed against the cancer. As a consequence, after treatment, patients may find themselves with both reduced amounts of cancer and a weakened immune system. Will this weakened immune protection recover and strengthen fast enough to hold off the small but still dangerous amounts of cancer?

Given that stress weakens the immune defenses, it would make sense that the development of more effective stress-coping skills could be of great importance to the cancer patient. How are these skills best taught to these patients?

Fortunately, there are a number of techniques now available for effective stress management. Among the most effective are progressive relaxation, autogenic training, meditation, cognitive therapy, and biofeedback. All of these techniques involve some degree of control of the body by the mind, whether directly—as in the case of progressive relaxation, autogenic training, and biofeedback—or indirectly—as with meditation and cognitive therapy.

Biofeedback

Approximately 15 years ago, a truly high-technology application to stress-related disorders was begun. Biofeedback is the electronic processing, quantification, and feedback, to the patient, of relevant physiological responses (Fuller, 1977). The technique can enhance quickly the ability of patients to be aware of strategies that are successful in producing antistress patterns. The biofeedback is usually an auditory or visual signal that is an analog of the actual biosignal. Thus, muscle tension can be converted into a tone, the frequency of which becomes proportionally higher as the degree of tension rises. Patients learn to keep the tone low by relaxing their muscles.

Progressive Relaxation, Autogenic
Training, and Systematic Desensitization

The objective, of course, is to produce a physiological pattern opposite to that
of the stress or "fight or flight" pattern. For over half a century both progressive relaxation and autogenic training have been used to do just that. Progressive relaxation involves the tensing and relaxing of the major muscle groups.
With continued training the patient learns to control smaller and smaller incre-
ments of tension. Progressive relaxation is particularly useful in developing a
patient's awareness of tension in the skeletal muscle system. Since the stress
pattern usually involves an increasing tonus in these muscles, an ability to relax
can counter much of the stress pattern effectively.

     Autogenic training, on the other hand, employs silent repetition of phrases
directed at the production of bodily sensations characteristic of a relaxed, antistress pattern. For example, the patient would repeat silently, "My right arm is
warm and heavy." This and other phrases are intended to produce sensations
that reflect muscle relaxation and an autonomic pattern of decreased sympathetic tonus.

     The development of this control requires a considerable amount of daily
practice. With both autogenic training and progressive relaxation the patient
must learn to become aware of the extremely subtle internal sensations that
signal the antistress pattern.

     At the Biofeedback Institute of Denver and the Cancer Self-Help Program
at Presbyterian Denver Hospital, patients practice at home with a cassette-tape
program. The sequence of training begins with an abbreviated form of progressive relaxation, then progresses to practice with autogenic exercises, followed by
a third phase incorporating systematic desensitization. Having learned to relax
under somewhat ideal conditions, the patients then must begin to transfer or
generalize the skill to everyday stressful situations. This is done through systematic desensitization, which is the behavior-therapy procedure in which a state
of relaxation is paired with the visualization of fearful situations. In this application, patients use their progressive relaxation and autogenically trained skills
to produce an antistress pattern as they visualize themselves in typical stressful
situations. A long history of research with systematic desensitization indicates
that the procedure does result in a decrease in fear in the actual situation.

     Our experience with approximately seven years of usage has convinced us
that the cassette-tape program constitutes a very successful stress management
program.

     Given that patients can be taught to relax and produce an antistress physi-
ological pattern, can they then transfer that skill to less-than-ideal situations?
For example, can patients stay reasonably relaxed while receiving radiation
therapy? By producing relaxation responses and visualizing the radiation as de-

stroying only the cancer, patients theoretically can decrease the immunosuppressive effects of the stress. Moreover, because patients take active rather than passive roles in the radiation procedure they in effect change the stress from "uncontrollable" to "controllable." Thus, patients produce an active coping response to the stress.

Patients can be taught to relax initially in the biofeedback training environment. After using biofeedback to guide themselves to a deep relaxation, they will visualize themselves in a variety of realistic stressful situations. Many of these situations will involve medical procedures; other stressful scenes may deal with work or family problems.

Each visualization is carried on until the biofeedback or a subjective feeling of anxiety indicates an increase of arousal. At this point the visualization is ended and relaxation is produced again. This sequence is repeated until patients can visualize each scene for at least one minute without appreciable increase in arousal. The transfer of relaxation responses to real-life situations tends to occur automatically after a short delay of perhaps a few days.

Imagery Procedures

After a person has learned to relax and has some experience of bodily control by using mental tools, the therapist may move on to suggest that these mental tools be applied directly to the cancer. Mental imagery, a way of visualizing the process of defeating the cancer, can be used regularly, not only to support patients' beliefs that they are participating actively in the treatment of the disease, but possibly to help stimulate their bodies toward health (Simonton & Matthews-Simonton, 1980).

This technique is actually not a new approach in medicine. Hypnosis, which relies heavily on the formation of mental images, long has been known to produce remarkable physical results. The rationale for daily relaxation and a lower level of arousal is well supported; however, the mechanisms by which imagery influences body systems to inhibit tumor progression are not well understood. The following brief description of the brain lateralization model is one influential explanation.

The Brain Lateralization
Model of Health/Illness

This model begins with the assertion that the two sides, or hemispheres, of the human brain control different functions. These are presented in Table 14-1. Note that the last functions listed are "conscious" on the left and "unconscious" on the right. Because few people can agree on a definition of conscious-

Table 14-1
Partial Listing of Cerebral Hemispheric Functions

Left	Right
Speech	Voice intonation contours
Language comprehension (abstract)	Language comprehension (concrete)
Logic	Emotion
Time sense (past, present, future)	Present oriented
Sequential (slow)	Parallel (fast)
Detail oriented	Gestalt oriented
Temporal	Spatial
Rhythm	Melody
Analytical aspects of mathematics (e.g., algebra)	Spatial aspects of mathematics (e.g., geometry)
Reason	Intuition
Convergent approach	Divergent approach
Relatively narrow arousal-level range over which it can function	Relatively wide arousal-level range over which it can function
Evolutionarily newer	Evolutionarily older
Conscious	Unconscious

ness, the differentiation remains somewhat ambiguous; however, our concepts of consciousness are closely tied to verbal ability, so it is more conventional to assume that the talkative, logical left hemisphere is the more conscious one.

Galin (1974), in an intriguing article, reviewed a great deal of the research on the functions of the cerebral hemispheres. He concluded that the functional description of right or nondominant hemisphere matched closely Freud's concept of the unconscious. Galin also mentioned that Ferenczi had noted that hysterical symptoms more often appeared on the left side of the body (the side controlled by the right hemisphere).

Galin, Diamond, and Braff (1977) verified Ferenczi's findings by examining conversion-reaction patients' records. Like Ferenczi, they found a significant tendency for the reactions to be lateralized on the left side of the body. This finding was reported independently by Stern (1977) and supports previous findings on the lateralization of symptoms classified as hypochondriacal (Kenyon, 1964).

Tucker (1981) concluded an exhaustive review of the research on lateral brain function and emotion with the statement, "The importance to emotion of the right hemisphere's cognitive functions suggests the possibility that right cortical regions may be particularly well connected with subcortical processes" (p. 22). This conclusion by Tucker is extremely important in light of the animal research previously reviewed which demonstrated how the subcortical structures, particularly the hypothalamus, are involved in immunosuppression (see also Stein, Keller, & Schleifer, 1981).

Let us assume for the moment that the right hemisphere indeed does have a greater influence than the left on subcortical functioning, particularly with regard to the more "negative" emotions. Perhaps we also may assume that the chronic generation of these emotions and the simultaneous inhibition of overt emotional behavior (i.e., keeping it inside) can result in immunosuppression. (Remember that it was the *uncontrollable* type of stress that increased cancer development in laboratory animals and correlated higher with illness than controllable stress in humans.) Thus, one could view health as somewhat delicately preserved—balanced on the tightrope of the immune system. Anything that weakens the system, even slightly, puts the individual in jeopardy. Uncontrollable, frustrating, chronic stress appears to be one such disrupting factor.

Interhemispheric Inhibition

As noted earlier, the inhibition of emotion may be one characteristic of the so-called "cancer personality." Brain lateralization research suggests that this could be an indication of inhibition of the right hemisphere by the left hemisphere. The right hemisphere can stimulate the emotional centers more easily. (Tucker, 1981) and in turn perhaps influence the immune system. In a general sense, we are taught to inhibit our emotional expression as a cultural phenomenon. The degree to which this inhibition is practiced in a culture may be related to cancer incidence. Consider information presented in Table 14-2, taken from the *World Health Statistics Annual 1977-1978* (1978). The incidence of cancer was compiled for 46 nations. We have shown the five highest and five lowest nations for incidence of cancer death in both males and females.

Table 14-2

Age-Adjusted Cancer Deaths per 100,000 Population, 1974-1975

	Ranking, 5 Highest-Incidence Countries	
	Males	*Females*
1	Czechoslovakia	Ireland
2	Scotland	Hungary
3	Belgium	Scotland
4	Hungary	Denmark
5	France	Austria
	Ranking, 5 Lowest Incidence Countries	
	Males	*Females*
42	Mexico	Panama
43	Philippines	Philippines
44	Dominican Republic	Honduras
45	Thailand	Dominican Republic
46	Honduras	Thailand

Source: *World Health Statistics Annual 1977-1978.*

The cultures represented in the high-incidence list differ from cultures in the low-incidence list with respect to such factors as climate, nutritional habits, and possibly the tendency to seek medical aid when ill. However, one also is struck by the difference between the high and low lists with regard to spontaneous expression of emotion. The cultures in the low-incidence list typically allow a greater degree of emotional freedom than those of the high-incidence list. One hypothesis suggests the minor (right) hemisphere may be less likely to initiate a weakening of the immune system when emotion is allowed expression a reasonable proportion of the time.

Conflict Between Hemispheres

It may be possible that highly civilized cultures unknowingly teach a degree of dominance of one hemisphere (the left) over the other (the right) such that conflict results due to the inability of the minor side to implement a psychophysiological program in conflict with the major side.

Is it even possible that the two sides could have conflicting programs? Might not the sequential, logical left consider a different approach to a problem situation than the fact-processing, emotional right? Galin (1974) states that "the two modes (holistic and analytic) may be in conflict; there seems to be some mutual antagonism between the analytic and the holistic."

Bogen and Bogen (1969) noted that "the possession of two independent problem-solving organs increases the prospects of a successful solution to a novel situation, although it has the hazard of conflict in the event of different solutions."

Galin (1974) has indicated that if a conflict occurs the left hemisphere seems to win control of the output channels most of the time. However, if the left is not able to "turn off" the right completely, it may "settle for" disconnecting the transfer of conflicting information from the right. Galin goes on to say that this cut-off mental process in the right hemisphere, not available to conscious thought, nevertheless may continue a life of its own. He further speculates that memory of the situation and its emotional concomitants and the frustrated plan of action all may persist, affecting subsequent perception and forming the basis for expectations and evaluations of future input.

The model we are proposing would go one step further and predict that certain of these frustrated plans may be implemented through somatic–autonomic pathways, as in hysterical conditions. However, we further speculate that the minor hemisphere may be able to produce a weakening of the immune system or initiate autoimmune reactions as a result of neural activity via the subcortical structures. The following list summarizes the logic of this model.

1. Stress and cancer are linked in most but not all studies.

2. Uncontrollable (inescapable) stress is implicated in immunosuppression.
3. Controllable (escapable) stress does not weaken, and may even strengthen, immune defense.
4. The hypothalamus is implicated in immunosuppression.
5. The hypothalamus, operating on trigger signals from the cortex and limbic system, directs much of the stress response and emotional behavior in general.
6. The right (or nondominant) cerebral hemisphere is more closely linked than the left to subcortical (emotional) structures such as the limbic system and the hypothalamus.
7. The right hemisphere appears to subserve the functions of the unconscious as described by Freud.
8. Conflict between hemispheres can occur when the two have opposing programs, action tendencies, or goals.
9. Right-brain, unconscious memories and action tendencies sometimes are prevented access to left-brain consciousness.
10. Thus, the right hemisphere could produce hysterical or conversion-reaction symptoms or immunosuppression or autoimmune reactions as a result of its "unconscious" programs.
11. These destructive programs cease when interhemispheric conflict is eliminated.
12. Conflict is minimized or eliminated when
    a. The left hemisphere program is changed to conform to right-hemisphere goals
    b. The right hemisphere program is changed to conform to left-hemisphere goals
    c. Change in the proper direction occurs in both left and right programs.

Application of the Model

Given that a conflict between cerebral hemispheres results in emotional and physical problems, a return to health should be facilitated better through a resolution of the conflict. It is further speculated that many of the conflicts arise because of scripts or programs generated in early childhood (perhaps prior to full maturation of the corpus callosum). It also is quite probable that many of these early scripts are repressed or in some way inaccessible to conscious retrieval attempts. In other words, they are stored in the right hemisphere, having been generated out of early *emotional* experiences, and are not fully accessible to the logical, left hemisphere.

The corpus callosum does not complete its myelinization until the eighth or ninth year of life. During this period, the left and right hemispheres are processing, each in their individual ways, all the raw data that enters the brain. Since the hemispheres process material in different ways (the left storing verbal information and converting input events into logical sequences; the right storing emotionally relative information such as facial and bodily configurations and tone of voice), we can begin to realize how easy it would be to store discrepant, conflicting scripts in the two hemispheres.

According to this speculative model, cancer development may be enhanced when there is a conflict between hemispheres and the nondominant program is chronically inhibited by the dominant hemisphere. Moreover, the ongoing dominant program, or coping style, *as perceived by the nondominant hemisphere,* is unsuccessful. These conflicts between hemispheres produce an uncomfortable psychological state. If this psychological state persists over a long period of time, it may lead to a physiological imbalance mediated by the right brain.

Changing Right-Brain Programs

Our left brain is a logical processor. If we feed in a good rationale for change, it probably will change. The right brain, however, doesn't process or appreciate logic. Its scripts are designed with emotional rather than logical language, so that a change in a right-brain script would likely be facilitated by an emotional procedure of some sort. Of course, when our emotions dominate, our right brain is active. There is some evidence that when our right brain is not dominating, it is difficult, if not impossible to change its script. Support for this idea comes from the extensive review on feeling and thinking by Zajonc (1980), who states that "the dismal failure in achieving substantial attitude change through various forms of communication or persuasion is another indication that affect is fairly independent and often impervious to cognition" (p. 158). Zajonc concludes that the apparent separation between affect and cognition may well have a psychological *and* a biological basis. In other words, if we stubbornly retain a left-brain dominance, the attempt to change a right-brain script will probably fail.

How, then, do we alter a right-brain (emotional) script? The technology for such a change is primitive and poorly researched at this point. Suffice it to say that some of the traditional modes of psychological intervention such as insight-oriented talking therapies or the use of pure behavioral change do not alter deep-seated, nonverbal, feeling-tone messages. It is only through the suspension of left-hemisphere dominance and accessing right-hemisphere functions that such a change occurs. Using relaxation techniques that lower one's level of arousal and loosen the left brain's narrow means of attending, combined with imagery that "speaks the language" of the right brain, we may elicit right-brain changes more effectively. Certainly, highly emotional psychotherapeutic techniques such as regression during reparenting may break through logical blocks and help restructure emotional programs.

In two pilot projects a combination of relaxation and mental imagery, biofeedback, psychotherapy, and emotional support as adjuncts to standard medical treatment have resulted in outcomes substantially different than those expected from standard treatment alone (Simonton et al., 1980; Gilbert et al., 1979). These preliminary outcomes, supported by the mass of laboratory and clinical data that piece together possible mechanisms to explain the observations, suggest further research in the area. This work points us toward an extension of medical oncology to include the study and treatment of psychobiological factors that may weigh heavily in the development and the progression of cancers.

References

Ader, R. *Psychoneuroimmunology*. New York: Academic Press, 1981.

Ader, R., & Cohen, N. Behaviorally conditioned immunosuppression. *Psychosomatic Medicine*, 1975, *37*, 333–340.

Amkraut, A., & Solomon, G. Stress and murine sarcoma virus (Maloney) induced tumors. *Cancer Research*, 1972, *32*, 1428–1433.

Amkraut, A., & Solomon, G. From the symbolic stimulus to the pathophysiologic response: Immune mechanisms. *International Journal of Psychiatry in Medicine*, 1975, *5*, 541–563.

Anisman, H. Neurochemical changes elicited by stress. In H. Anisman & G. Bignami (Eds.), *Psychopharmacology of Assertively Motivated Behavior*. New York: Plenum Press, 1978.

Anisman, H., Pizzino, A., & Sklar, L. Coping with stress, norepinephrine depletion and escape performance. *Brain Research*, 1980, *191*, 583–588.

Bahnson, C., & Bahnson, M. Denial and repression of primitive impulses and of disturbing emotions in patient, with malignant neoplasms. In D. Kissen & L. LeShan (Eds.), *Psychosomatic Aspects of Neoplastic Disease*. London: Pitman, 1964.

Bartrop, R., Lazarus, L., Luckhurst, E., Kiloh, L., & Penny, R. Depressed lymphocyte function after bereavement. *Lancet*, 1977, *1*, 834–836.

Bieliauskas, L., Shekelle, R., Garron, D., Maliza, C., Ostfeld, A., Paul, O., & Raynor, W. Psychological depression and cancer mortality. Paper presented at the annual meeting of the American Psychosomatic Society, Dallas, Texas, 1979.

Bogen, J., & Bogen, G. The other side of the brain, III: The corpus callosum and creativity. *Bulletin of Los Angeles Neurology Society*, 1969, *34*, 191–220.

Cherek, D., Lane, J., Freeman, M., & Smith, J. Receptor changes following shock avoidance. *Society of Neurosciences Abstracts*, 1980, *6*, 543.

Dechambre, R., & Gosse, C. Individual versus group caging of mice with grafted tumors. *Cancer Research*, 1973, *33*, 140–144.

Derogatis, L., Abeloff, M., & Melisaratos, N. Psychological coping mechanisms and survival time in metastatic breast cancer. *Journal of the American Medical Association*, 1979, *242*, 1504–1508.

Doll, R. Strategy for detection of cancer hazards in man. *Nature,* 1977, *265,* 589–596.

Fox, B. Premorbid psychological factors as related to cancer incidence. *Journal of Behavioral Medicine,* 1978, *1,* 45–133.

Frank, J. *Persuasion and Healing.* New York: Schocken Books, 1974.

Furth, J. Hormones as etiological agents in neoplasia. In F. F. Becker (Ed.), *Cancer: A Comprehensive Treatise* (Vol. 1). New York: Plenum Press, 1975.

Galin, D. Implications for psychiatry of left and right cerebral specialization. *Archives of General Psychiatry,* 1974, *31,* 572–583.

Galin, D., Diamond, R., & Braff, D. Lateralization of conversion symptoms: More frequent on the left. *American Journal of Psychiatry,* 1977, *134,* 578–580.

Gilbert, E., Miller, J., Gilbert, J., Budzynski, T., & Bernton, T. Psychological intervention and its effect on longevity in cancer patients: A pilot study. *International Journal of Radiation Oncology,* 1979, suppl. no. 2, 87.

Goldstein, M., & Nakajima, K. The effect of disulfiram on the biosynthesis of catecholamines during exposure of rats to cold. *Life Sciences,* 1966, *5,* 175–179.

Gordon, R., Spector, S., Sjoerdsma, A., & Vdenfriend, S. Increased synthesis of norepinephrine and epinephrine in the intact rat during exercise and exposure to cold. *Journal of Pharmacology and Experimental Therapeutics,* 166, *153,* 440–447.

Greer, S. Psychological consequences of cancer. *Practitioner,* 1979, *222,* 173–178.

Holden, C. Behavioral medicine: An emergent field. *Science,* 1980, *209,* 479.

Horne, R., & Picard, R. Psychosocial risk factors for lung cancer. *Psychosomatic Medicine,* 1979, *41,* 503–514.

Huggins, C. Endocrine-induced regression of cancers. *Science,* 1967, *156,* 1050–1054.

Kenyon, F. Hypochondriasis: A clinical study. *British Journal of Psychiatry,* 1964, *110,* 478–488.

Kissen, D. Present status of psychosomatic cancer research. *Geriatrics,* 1969, *24,* 129.

Kissen, D. Psychosocial factors, personality and prevention of lung cancer. *Medical Officer,* 1966, *116,* 135–138.

Klein, G. Immunological surveillance against neoplasia. *The Harvey Lectures,* 1973–1974, Series 69, 71–102.

LeShan, L. Psychological states as factors in the development of malignant disease: A critical review. *Journal of the National Cancer Institute.* 1959, *22,* 1–18.

LeShan, L. An emotional life-history pattern associated with neoplastic disease. *Annals of the New York Academy of Sciences,* 1966, *125,* 780–793.

Nagao, M., Sugimura, T., & Matsushima, T. Environmental mutagens and carcinogens. In H. L. Roman, A. Campbell, & L. M. Dandler (Eds.), *Annual Review of Genetics* (Vol. 12). Palo Alto, Calif.: Annual Reviews, 1978.

Newberry, B., Frankie, G., Beatty, P., Maloney, B., & Gilchrist, J. Shock stress and DMBA-induced mammary tumors. *Psychosomatic Medicine,* 1972, *34,* 295–303.

Newberry, B., Gildow, J., Wogan, J., & Reese, R. Inhibition of Huggins tumors by forced restraint. *Psychosomatic Medicine*, 1976, *38*, 155-162.

New York Academy of Sciences. *Annals of the New York Academy of Sciences*, 1966, *125*, entire issue.

New York Academy of Sciences. *Annals of the New York Academy of Sciences*, 1969, *164*, entire issue.

Pradham, S., and Ray, P. Effects of stress on growth of transplanted and 7, 12-dimethylbenz (a) anthracene-induced tumors and their modification by psychotropic drugs. *Journal of the National Cancer Institute*, 1974, *53*, 1241-1245.

Ray, P., & Pradham, S. Growth of transplanted and induced tumors in rats under a schedule of punished behavior. *Journal of the National Cancer Institute*, 1974, *52*, 575-577.

Riley, V. Psychoneuroendocrine influences on immunocompetence and neoplasia. *Science*, 1981, *212*, 1100-1109.

Rogentine, N., Van Kammen, D., Fox, B., Docherty, J., Rosenblatt, J., Boyd, S., & Bunney, W. Psychological factors in prognosis of malignant melanoma: A prospective study. *Psychosomatic Medicine*, 1979, *41*, 147-164.

Rogers, M., Dubey, D., & Reich, P. The influence of the psyche and the brain on immunity and disease susceptibility: A critical review. *Psychosomatic Medicine*, 1979, *41*, 147-164.

Saarela, S., Hissa, R., Hohtola, E., & Jorenen, E. Effect of a-methyl-paratyrosine and temperature stress on monoamine and metabolite levels in the pigeon. *Journal of Thermal Biology*, 1977, *2*, 121-129.

Schmale, A., & Iker, H. The psychological setting of uterine cervical cancer. *Annals of the New York Academy of Sciences*, 1966, *125*, 807-813.

Schwartz, G. Psychobiological foundations of psychotherapy and behavior change. In S. Garfield & A. Bergin (Eds.), *Handbook of Psychotherapy and Behavior Change* (2nd ed.). New York: John Wiley, 1978.

Selye, H. *The Stress of Life*. New York: McGraw-Hill, 1956.

Simmonds, M. Effects of environmental temperature on the turnover of noradrenaline in hypothalamus and other areas of the rat brain. *Journal of Physiology* (London), 1969, *203*, 199-210.

Simonton, O., & Matthews-Simonton, S. *Getting Well Again*. New York: Bantam, 1980.

Simonton, O., Matthews-Simonton, S., & Sparks, T. Psychological intervention in the treatment of cancer. *Psychosomatics*, 1980, *21*, 226-233.

Sklar, L., & Anisman, H. Stress and coping factors influence tumor growth. *Science*, 1979, *205*, 513-515.

Sklar, L., & Anisman, H. Social stress influences tumor growth. *Psychosomatic Medicine*, 1980, *42*, 347-365.

Sklar, L., & Anisman, H. Stress and cancer. *Psychological Bulletin*, 1981, *89*, 369-407.

Solomon, G., Levine, S., & Kraft, J. Early experience and immunity. *Nature*, 1969, *220*, 821-822.

Stein, M., Keller, S., & Schleifer, S. The hypothalamus and the immune response. In H. Weiner, M. Hofer, & A. Stonkard (Eds.), *Brain, Behavior and Bodily Disease*. New York: Raven Press, 1981.

Stern, D. Handedness and the lateral distribution of conversion reactions. *Journal of Nervous and Mental Disease*, 1977, *164*, 122-128.

Stolk, J., Conner, R., Levine, S., & Barchas, J. Brain norepinephrine metabolism and shock-induced fighting behavior in rats: Differential effects of shock and fighting on the neurochemical response to a common footshock stimulus. *Journal of Pharmacology and Experimental Therapeutics*, 1974, *190*, 193-209.

Stone, E. Stress and catecholamines. In A. Friedhoff (Ed.), *Catecholamines and Behavior* (Vol. 2), New York: Plenum Press, 1975.

Storer, J. B. Radiation carcinogenesis. In F. F. Becker (Ed.), *Cancer: A Comprehensive treatise* (Vol. 1). New York: Plenum Press, 1975.

Thomas, C., & Duszynski, K. Closeness to parents and the family constellation in a prospective study of five disease states: Suicide, mental illness, malignant tumor, hypertension and coronary artery disease. *Johns Hopkins Medical Journal*, 1974, *134*, 251-270.

Tucker, D. Lateral brain function, emotion, and conceptualization. *Psychological Bulletin*, 1981, *89*, 19-46.

Upton, A. C. Physical carcinogenesis: Radiation—history and source. In F. F. Becker (Ed.), *Cancer: A Comprehensive Treatise* (Vol. 1). New York: Plenum Press, 1975.

Visintainer, M., Volpicelli, J., & Seligman, M. Tumor rejection in rats after inescapable or escapable shock. *Science*, 1982, *216*, 437-439.

Weiss, J. Effects of coping behavior with and without a feedback signal on stress pathology in rats. *Journal of Comparative and Physiological Psychology*, 1971, *77*, 1-13, 22-30.

Weiss, J., Glazer, H., & Pohorecky, L. Coping behavior and neurochemical changes: An alternative for the origin of "learned helplessness" experiments. In G. Serban & A. Kling (Ed.), *Animal Models in Human Psychobiology*. New York: Plenum Press, 1976.

Weiss, J., Pohorecky, L., Salman, S., & Gruenthal, M. Attenuation of gastric lesions by psychological aspects of aggression in rats. *Journal of Comparative and Physiological Psychology*, 1976, *90*, 252-259.

Weiss, J., Stone, E., & Harrell, N. Coping behavior and brain norepinephrine levels in rats. *Journal of Comparative and Physiological Psychology*, 1970, *72*, 153-160.

Welsch, C., & Nagasawa, H. Prolactin and murine mammary tumorogenesis: A review. *Cancer Research*, 1977, *37*, 951-963.

World Health Statistics Annual 1977-1978, Vol. 1, 1978.

Zajonc, R. Feeling and thinking: Preferences need no inferences. *American Psychologist*, 1980, *35*, 176-186.

15

A Plea for Humanism

Yvonne Fotes

In September 1978, my daughter had her first biopsy and bone marrow test performed in our small hometown hospital. These tests were sent away for analysis, and the three weeks that followed while we awaited the results seemed endless. We filled those days with living: boating, hiking, and dangling our feet in crystal-clear streams. We seemed to have a special appreciation for sunny days, and we soaked in our beautiful scenery. We celebrated Kim's seventeenth birthday with a party. Kim continued working, and both she and her sister started the new school year.

About four months later Kim asked me if I hadn't been scared about the tests. I said, "Yes, I was terrified." I expected to hear that I had really blown it, but Kim said, "I knew you were, but they were good weeks in spite of the tests and I'm glad we had them. Thanks for not taking them away from me, but for making them the very best that they could be."

Kim was a beautiful, pudgy, and adorable baby. Before Kim entered junior high school she had attended six different schools because her father changed jobs several times. She managed quite well and truly seemed to believe that a house was just a house, but the family made it a home.

Kim was happiest when she spent time on her grandparents' ranch. She was given her first pony at three and would spend subsequent summers on the ranch riding and working with the horses. Everyone knew that, to stay on grandpa's good side, one had only to love his granddaughter and agree with him that she was delightful. Grandpa called her his "foreman," and she was not only the smallest, but probably the most loyal and dedicated foreman he ever had. As time passed, she became a very competent and capable horsewoman. The entire town spoiled Kim, as they had spoiled her mother in earlier years. I'm sure her grandparents, the ranch, and the town contributed much to Kim's good self-image. She had much respect for older people and thoroughly enjoyed conversation with them. Many have said that she never walked by without saying "hello" and acknowledging them. She was assertive and didn't hesitate to ask questions.

Kim shared her life with her red-headed sister, who was three and one-half years younger than she. Her sister quickly gained the nickname "Me Too," because the greatest part of her day consisted of trying to keep up with Kim. It was a typical sister relationship. There were merry-go-rounds, rainbows, cotton candy, sticky kisses, and camaraderie in battles of self-defense when Mom was on the warpath. As time went on, the loyalty and pride they developed for one another was boundless. I wish it could have lasted longer.

After 19 years of marriage, Kim's father and I separated. This deeply hurt Kim, as it was a very painful and heartbreaking experience for an idealistic girl of sixteen. During the divorce settlement, we could make no future plans, and we lived for eight months with wall-to-wall packed boxes. Financially, as well as emotionally, life was in shambles. We were fortunate to have close friends during this time. Our attorney was truly a blessing to us, for he not only was honest, dedicated, and courageous, but he was compassionate and caring. He was to remain in our lives about eight months, and in the end he put many pieces together from which we rebuilt our future. We even unpacked. Perhaps as a consequence of this man's efforts and concerns, Kim developed the desire to become an attorney.

In August 1978 Kim went to a dermatologist regarding a very small blemish above her eye. He said it was nothing but to return in a month. When she returned, she was referred to an ear, nose, and throat specialist, as the blemish had evolved into a bump. The ENT specialist decided to watch it as it had decreased in size since her visit to the dermatologist. By the next appointment, the bump had grown larger and the decision to biopsy the mass was made. The night before Kim was to enter the hospital, she noticed a similar bump on her abdomen and another on her arm. In terror, I called the doctor and told him the news. The next day he performed a biopsy of the mass on her arm. While Kim was in surgery someone brought me a slip requesting permission for Kim to have a bone marrow test. I signed it with trembling hands, many tears, and an aching heart. Suddenly the bright, hopeful future looked grim and ominous.

We waited for weeks for the test results, and when they did not come, our physician made arrangements for Kim to enter an out-of-state hospital. That hospital stay lasted one month, and tests performed during that time confirmed the diagnosis of lymphoma.

During Kim's care in Denver, she always was treated as a person, with love. She was allowed to be brave, to be scared, to be angry, to be hopeful, and to be sick. One day when her primary doctor was out of town, she refused to allow a biopsy to be performed on her face. It developed into a difficult "stand-off," as her doctor had left orders for the biopsy. It ended with the doctors retreating. I did not scold her, because I felt she had the right to question and to say no, after listening to the facts. As much as I loved her, I knew that she and she alone would be the one to endure. When her primary doctor returned, he agreed that a biopsy could be done on another tumor, and radiation could resolve the tumor on her face. This incident was of critical importance. Kim still had the right to be the decision maker in matters regarding her own body. It should be noted that the doctors remained her friends and did not make her refusal a personal issue or use it to label her. When I first met her primary doctor he said, "We treat the total little girl, not just the sickness." Later he would say, "We listen to the patient." At the time it simply sounded like plain old-fashioned common sense. It did not seem like a medical issue. It would be three months later before I fully realized the ramifications of such a basically simple statement.

During that month Kim received extensive tests, radiation, and her first chemotherapy treatment. The chemotherapy made her violently ill, but it was decided that she should return home when she felt better, in hopes that she could continue school while receiving chemotherapy and radiation treatments.

When we got back home, Kim did return to school. With all of her determination mustered, she shopped for an outfit "appropriate" for senior pictures. The beaming smile in the pictures belied the fact that she'd been in the hospital a month. The day the pictures were taken will never be forgotten. That night her hair fell out in clumps. I wish I could have shared her courage and her heartaches in dealing with her friends and teachers. There were many beautiful friends and supporters, but there also were threads of failure in finding understanding and knots of loneliness and rejection.

I'd like you to picture a girl who had known heartache and sorrow—a girl who, until her sickness, was filled with vitality, potential, and, yes, dreams. Then try to picture what her emotions must have been. The fear, the devastating fear. The panic. The anger of, "Why me, God?" The creeping realization that life was becoming more and more limited, and this was *Senior* year. And finally the loss of her crowning glory, her beautiful hair. I can still hear the sobs, feel the heartache, and see the anger as her hair came tumbling down and mingled with her falling tears. She was inconsolable. The words I offered fell on deaf ears, and in despair my tears joined hers. This was only the beginning of the suffering and devastation which was to come.

With chemotherapy it was not uncommon for Kim to vomit every 15 minutes through the night and until noon the next day. The nightmare of the dreaded therapy increased her depression immensely. About two to three days prior to chemotherapy, her emotions would go into a tailspin. I would take her to the hospital as soon as I got off work on Friday afternoons. That way she could receive chemotherapy on Friday and I could stay with her through the weekend. I wish I could convey the anguish that consumed me as I watched her nightmare. I reached the point where I'd walk to the car crying. I'd sob on the drive home from work, then stop about two blocks away from our house. I'd blow my nose, apply my makeup, try to bring positive thoughts to mind, and then pick up my daughter for the drive to the hospital. When I think of my personal anguish during this time, I know it must have been magnified a hundred times for my daughter, as she was the one who endured the treatments.

Aside from the anguish and illness that chemotherapy caused, it was my daughter's only hope. Maybe chemotherapy could control those cancer cells. Go for it, fight for it. Some win, some lose, and, yes, Kim was a fighter. Once a doctor told her, "You don't have to go through with this," and he walked out of the room. But Kim realized it was her only lifeline, and in tears she said, "Wrong: it's the only choice I have if I want to live." I had to agree with her.

By this time, it had become painfully clear that a drastic change in attitude had taken place among the doctors and other medical staff at our hometown hospital. The first time Kim had gone in, for the initial testing, the hospital staff had seemed warm and kind. Then we went to Denver, where Kim also was treated with caring and respect. But when we returned home, things were very different. I've asked myself over and over what caused the change. Kim was still polite and considerate. She was still Kim, *but* this time with a lymphoma. Was that the difference? Were the medical professionals trying to isolate themselves from Kim and her feelings? Was the price of humanism too high? Were they not trained well enough to deal with the monster disease, cancer? Was it because they were not trained to talk with skill, comfort, and concern to a 17-year-old cancer patient? In Denver I was to meet other teenagers with cancer. They all missed home a great deal, but some had similar negative experiences and did not want to return to their hometown hospitals. There must be a need for better or broader training in some regions. I wish with my whole heart that I had a smooth, sophisticated means of conveying the tremendous need for a renewed interest in humanism in the hospitals not connected with research and treatment centers. I don't. I can only share a bit more of a very, very painful time in our lives.

At the research center it took about 30 minutes to administer chemotherapy. In our hometown the same chemotherapy that Kim received took three and one-half hours. Please consider the agony of this sort of situation. In one instance it took the nurse over five times to start an I.V.; Kim lost her patience and began swearing, not a usual response for her. The nurse apologized and gave a little sermon on how everyone needs to learn. The nurse was not new to her job, and, ironically, the vein she eventually was successful in entering was the one Kim had asked her to use in the first place. Perhaps a patient with a short-term illness who is going to be hospitalized briefly and then return to a normal, healthy life should have more patience. However, a patient with cancer, who has faced endless needles and pain and for whom the future holds only more of the same, should not be subjected to incompetency in the name of inexperience. For the most part, no one seemed to pay attention or care if the I.V. infiltrated. Kim did. I did.

Our small-town hospital was often dirty and always filled with "hospital odors." Kim was placed in a room with a retarded woman of about 20 who required diapers. When the diapers were changed, they were thrown in a waste-basket next to my daughter's bed. I asked that they please be removed from the room as the stench was unbearable to my daughter, who was already violently ill from the chemotherapy. After persistent requests I finally resorted to setting the wastebasket in the hall myself, after the diapers had been placed in it. I felt this situation was another example of general inconsideration.

On my daughter's last stay in our hospital, when she was so sick during an endless night, a young nurse said out loud, "I wonder how it feels to be so young and to be dying." Kim cried. It was relatively early in her fight, and while she definitely knew the odds, she was fighting for time and a possible remission. One of the things for which I am most grateful to the Denver medical center staff is that they, unlike our local professionals, didn't bury my daughter before she died. Often with cancer, people pull back and avoid involvement with the patient. Never once to my knowledge did Kim say, "Cure me." She would say, "What are we going to do now? What about the pain? Can't we do anything for the nausea?" I, as well as Kim, desperately needed to know that someone cared enough to be there, to offer us some form of help or relief. I remember talking to one doctor in nuclear medicine. When I asked if it wasn't hard working with cancer patients, he said, "No; they demand nothing." I didn't respond. I couldn't comprehend his statement. Perhaps older patients don't demand; perhaps they lie quietly waiting to die. If they are comfortable with that, then it is their right. But I believe one has the right to demand. Again I thought of the kind doctor who said, "We treat the total little girl."

Probably the next situation was a problem unique to our hometown, where there are two hospitals. As I understand it, the records from one hospital are stored at the other hospital, and, because the one hospital did not have the records, Kim was asked the same questions each time she was admitted. Most of the questions were not pertinent. Most of them were painful to my daughter. The person asking the questions had no finesse, nor even knowledge of the correct terminology. In fact, my daughter spelled many of the words for her. Because they were unfamiliar with the diagnosis, the staff said, "Show me your cancer." Never did they use the word tumor, and seldom did they use the word please. They did not seem to comprehend that there were tumors throughout my daughter's body, internally as well as externally, I wish I had the ability to describe the scene. I can still see the expression on my poor little girl's face. I asked if they couldn't get the records prior to her admission; would they please let me pick them up. The answer was, "No, we can't allow you to do that because of policy." There is no way I can condone policy of this type. My daughter is dead, the records exist, and I'm sure that their value is not worth the pain that they caused her.

Another time my daughter had been in terrible pain, on strong pain medication for at least four days. Arrangements had been made several days in advance for her hospital admittance. She was anxious to enter the hospital, hoping that the chemotherapy would attack the tumor and relieve her suffering. She had been crawling because it was too painful to walk. We arrived to be told that there was no available space. My daughter cried as we sat in the waiting room. Eventually, another teenage girl walked out, against medical advice, and my daughter got her room. Once again the feeling conveyed was, "You don't matter!" By contrast, in Denver, Kim once was admitted to the hospital a day prior to treatment, to be assured of a bed. Another time her release was delayed because a storm had come up and they did not want her out in it. Did it upset her? No; it said to her, "We're here. We care."

My daughter usually received chemotherapy between one and one-half and two hours after entering our local hospital. On these days, she ate very little, omitting evening meals because of the terrible nausea. Once she was admitted around 5:30 P.M., and by 9:30 she still hadn't received her chemotherapy. Kim asked when she would receive chemotherapy and was told that the doctor had not yet placed the orders. Hearing that, my daughter threw herself in the corner of the bed against the wall and cried hysterically. I can still hear her sobbing, "I wish I were dead." No one, myself included, could calm her. Finally, I suggested she call the doctor and talk with him. I think that the suggestion restored her sense of power, the sense that she had the right to know what and when something would be done for her. She quit crying, called, and firmly asked him please to place the orders and to inform her of when she was to receive chemotherapy. He did as he was asked but said he did not realize that time was of importance to her. This doctor had no rapport with my daughter. Perhaps Kim's age was something with which he could not cope. Perhaps there was simply a personality clash. If there had been another oncologist in town, we would have changed doctors; as it was, we were stuck in a bad situation. It is interesting that on the medical report I carried by hand to Denver he had labeled my daughter as "hostile."

During that time Kim and I had felt extreme fear, panic, and total isolation. We learned firsthand the meaning of dehumanization. It seemed that, all along, my daughter was perceived more and more as an object than a human being. I deeply regret the times I remained much too passive. I also feel there were times when I was written off as emotional and an overly protective mother. I think both my daughter and I were looked upon as complainers who didn't understand medical procedure. Their attitude was, "Let them talk and complain, but we don't need to listen." I wonder if they thought Kim was going through a "stage" and that she was reacting just as dying patients are supposed to. I believe we live continually in stages, both in sickness and in health. I do not believe that terminally ill patients progress like clockwork through neat stages. I think the concept of stages can be very dangerous if it is used to simply label, categorize, and dismiss patients. This releases the need for in-depth understanding of patients and their individual needs.

Christmas was upon us. The tree, a gift from friends, was perfect. The holy crib was in place, and the tradition-worn stocking was hung as usual. Somehow my stubborn Kim had forced herself to shop. Each gift was special and a keepsake intended to last our lifetime. Kim wanted to go to Midnight Mass as we'd always done. Her sister and grandmother went an hour early to save a special pew. Kim, her grandfather, a special friend, and myself went just as Mass was beginning. I'll always remember her beautiful, radiant face as she joined in singing every hymn. Because of her tremendous spirit, Kim lived through Christmas.

The day after Christmas we flew to Denver. As the stars twinkled overhead we toasted one another with champagne. Kim giggled delightfully and we talked of past occasions and of things to come. We looked like a twosome on a seasonal holiday. We weren't. Kim would never return home.

As we walked into the hospital it was like a homecoming. Everyone on the floor rushed to see, greet, and hug Kim. As word spread that Kim was back, people from different floors came to visit. Kim and I both knew that we were no longer alone. Even as an outpatient Kim would return to the floor to say hi and to soak in warmth and kindness.

At the Denver hospital a nurse asked me for additional background on Kim, including whether anything in particular annoyed her. I gave some personal background; she loved horses, singing, and was an "A" student. She happened to hate the smell of alcohol, which sometimes made her sick. Thoughtfully, they used an alcohol substitute. One doctor asked if there was anything she liked to eat after chemotherapy. In the middle of winter, with a tremendously hectic schedule, her doctor managed to shop for her, and the next morning Kim received a brown bag from him, with a watermelon inside. She was delighted, and ate it with a vigorous appetite. When he was out of town, this same doctor called about her condition. He treated her spirit and her soul, and he will never be forgotten.

After surviving a bone-marrow rescue, Kim was told that she would have to receive chemotherapy weekly. She received massive doses of chemotherapy and additional ineffective nausea medications. As I watched my beautiful little girl in pain, violently ill to her stomach, I began to feel numb. At times it seemed as if the room were spinning. I wanted to cry out for help, but I knew there was nothing more that could be done; the world continued spinning: anguish, helplessness, despair, spinning-spinning-spinning.

Then a door suddenly opened. Life again had value. There were fancy restaurants, which Kim adored. She enjoyed shrimp, lobster, and steak. She attacked fried mushrooms, pizza, hamburgers, and Mom's home cooking. I can still hear the shared laughter as a cherry in the whipped cream trickled off the side of a huge sundae. There was even some shopping and a little dancing. There were movies, a basketball game, and attendance at a beloved ballet. It was good. It was a new humane medicine, tetrahydrocannabinol (THC), which dramatically decreased Kim's nausea and vomiting from chemotherapy. I found a rough draft of a letter Kim had written to Dr. Garb, who was responsible for giving her THC. I share it with the hope that research will continue to search for newer and better methods for improving the quality of life.

Thank you for allowing me to receive THC. The difference between taking chemo without THC and with the THC is tremendous. I'm so grateful for the relief it gave me.

Chemotherapy, in my case, is effective. It seems to kill the cancer cells and I feel extremely encouraged as to my eventual recovery. However, chemotherapy does much more than kill the deadly cells. It kills some of the good cells, and, worst of all, it makes me violently ill. Just the thought of chemotherapy turns my stomach, and, in agony, I ask myself: How much more can I take? Is it worth it? The constant fight against cancer is a steep climb, and when coupled with medications which succeed in making me feel worse than before, the fight sometimes seems pointless. In my particular fight, I have no room for doubts. Doubts send me into a frightening sea of devastation.

After experiencing THC, I feel deeply relieved. Here is a medication that enables me to walk to the hospital week after week for treatments, with the knowledge that this time I can feel a hundred percent more positive and determined; feelings so important. For example, after my last chemo with THC, I was able to attend my cousin's basketball game the following evening. In the past, without THC, it was at least a week before I could resume a "normal" life.

I would like to return home; we've been gone for more than a month and I miss it more each day. Yet the thought of receiving chemotherapy without the THC sends me once again into the frightening sea I mentioned earlier. I'm hoping that I will be able to return home with THC and continue the treatments. The answer to my question, "How much more pain can I endure?" is unfortunately, "Not much." It is with great appreciation for your understanding that I close.

Throughout my daughter's last days in Denver, we received only kindness and care. Her primary doctor never left town without giving us a phone number; we always could reach him. Even when he couldn't do something medically for Kim, he frequently would stop, visit, and listen.

At the Denver hospital everyone wanted to see Kim doing the things that teenagers do. With all the pain and heartache, my little girl again had moments of laughter and sunshine. The many good and kind deeds performed for my daughter and myself could fill a book. Doctors and nurses came to visit my little girl on their days off. They brought her flowers, gifts, and friendship. They had a pizza party. There was a guitar and beloved music. On coffee breaks people from all over the hospital came to visit her. I have a number of letters commenting on my daughter's love for life and for her courage. There are letters expressing how much she taught them and how she will never be forgotten. I feel obligated to mention these acts, as it was obvious that once she found understanding and professionalism in these people she quickly gave her heart and won theirs. They never accused her of being "hostile!"

The day my daughter died, the hospital room quietly filled and there wasn't a dry eye. I hope those dear people will always have the courage to continue to care. I hope they feel joy and pride in their work. I hope they can remember the smiles and giggles that would not have been possible without them. As I wept and packed Kim's belongings I remembered my daughter telling her grandparents, "These aren't just doctors and nurses, these are my friends." I give thanks for the wonderful people who were part of our lives, for in them we truly found the meaning of the word "humanism."

Index

Index